WALL PILATES

Workout for Women

▶▷▶▷ Guided Exercise Routines with Illustrations to Sculpt, Strengthen, and Tone Your Muscles and Body

By
Sarah Mckenzie

© Copyright 2023 by Sarah Mckenzie - All rights reserved.

This document is geared towards providing exact and reliable information in regard to the topic and issue covered. The publication is sold with the idea that the publisher is not required to render accounting, officially permitted, or otherwise, qualified services. If advice is necessary, legal or professional, a practiced individual in the profession should be ordered.

From a Declaration of Principles which was accepted and approved equally by a Committee of the American Bar Association and a Committee of Publishers and Associations. In no way is it legal to reproduce, duplicate, or transmit any part of this document in either electronic means or in printed format. Recording of this publication is strictly prohibited, and any storage of this document is not allowed unless with written permission from the publisher. All rights reserved.

The information provided herein is stated to be truthful and consistent, in that any liability, in terms of inattention or otherwise, by any usage or abuse of any policies, processes, or directions contained within is the solitary and utter responsibility of the recipient reader. Under no circumstances will any legal responsibility or blame be held against the publisher for any reparation, damages, or monetary loss due to the information herein, either directly or indirectly.

Respective authors own all copyrights not held by the publisher. The information herein is offered for informational purposes solely and is universal as such. The presentation of the information is without a contract or any type of guaranteed assurance. The trademarks that are used are without any consent, and the publication of the trademark is without permission or backing by the trademark owner. All trademarks and brands within this book are for clarifying purposes only and are owned by the owners themselves, not affiliated with this document.

YOUR FREE GIFT

As a way of saying thanks for your purchase,
I'm offering **"The Wall Pilates Fit Journal"** for **FREE** to you!

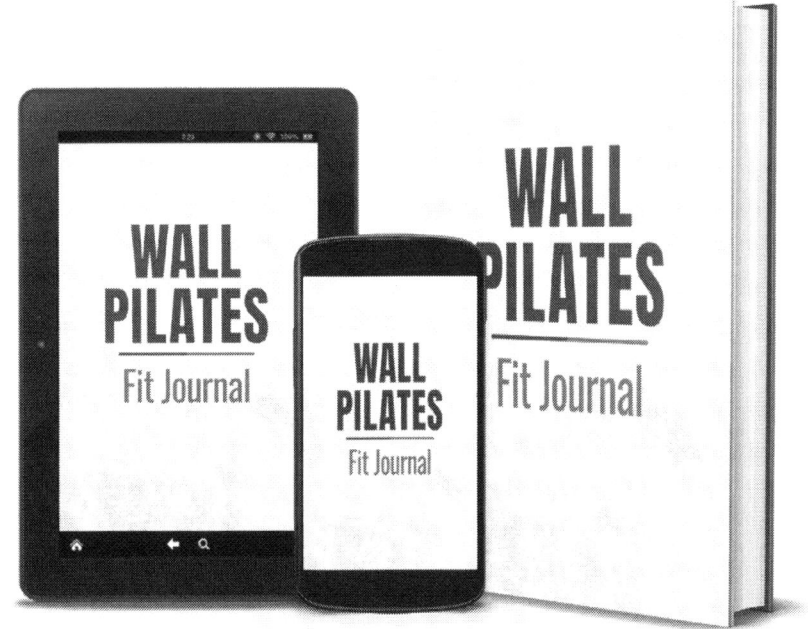

Here is a tiny fraction of what you will find inside:

- Measurements Tracking
- Weekly Fitness Tracking
- Daily Fitness Tracking

SCAN THE QR CODE AND GET YOUR GIFT!

TABLE OF CONTENTS

WORKOUTS FLOWS	5
INTRODUCTION	11
Is Wall Pilates for You?	12
The Genesis of Pilates: A Brief History	13
Reasons Pilates is For You	13
CHAPTER 1. WHY WALL PILATES	15
Benefits of Pilates	17
Yoga vs. Pilates: Unveiling the Differences and Common Ground	19
HIIT vs. Pilates: Unpacking the Contrasts and Synergies	20
Now, What Should You Choose?	22
CHAPTER 2. BEFORE YOU START	25
A List of All You Need	26
Your Mindset	26
CHAPTER 3. ACHIEVING TONE ABS	29
Workouts	30
CHAPTER 4: IMPROVING BACK POSTURE	45
Workouts	46
CHAPTER 5. SHAPING THE BUTTOCKS	59
Workouts	60
CHAPTER 6. FITNESS TRACKER	73
Fitness Plans for the Month	75
CHAPTER 7. EATING THE RIGHT NUTRITION	79
Bonus Recipes	81
CONCLUSION	96

WORKOUTS FLOWS

▶▶▶▶ ACHIEVING TONE ABS - WORKOUTS

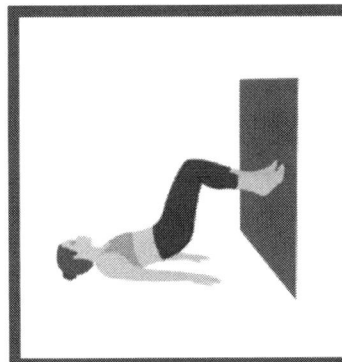
BRIDGE RAISES
PAG. 30

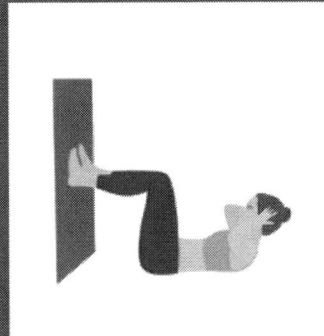
CRUNCHES
PAG. 31

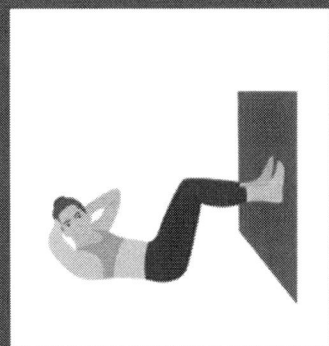
CRUNCH TWISTER
PAG. 32

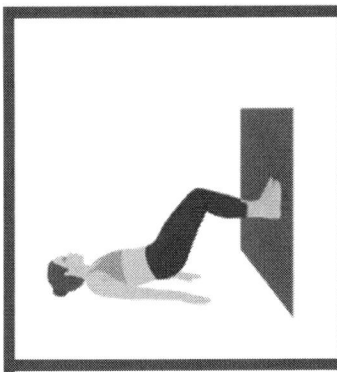
BRIDGE KNEE TO CHEST
PAG. 33

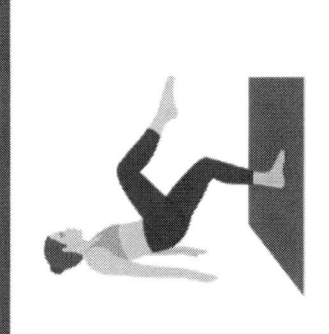
ONE-LEG BRIDGE RAISE
PAG. 34

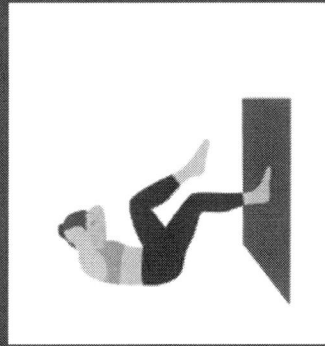
KNEE TO CHEST
PAG. 35

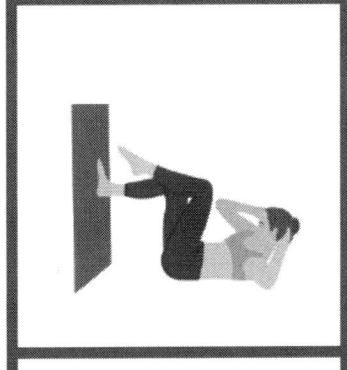
OPPOSITE KNEE TO ELBOW
PAG. 36

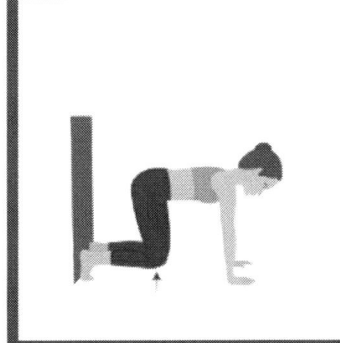
3-SECOND BEAR CRAWL
PAG. 37

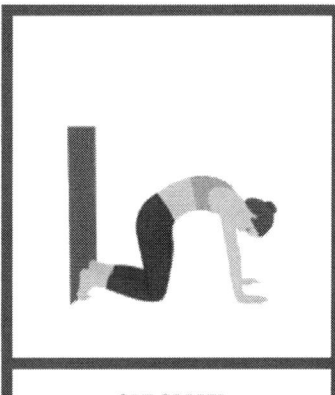
CAT-CAMEL
PAG. 39

▶▶▶▶ ACHIEVING TONE ABS - WORKOUTS

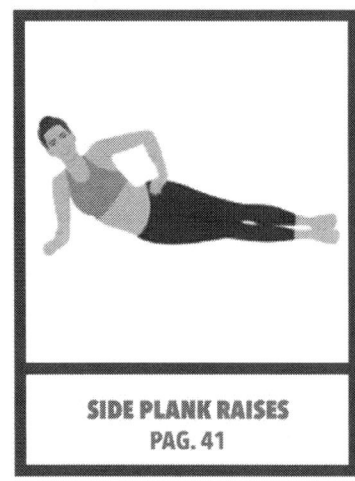

SIDE PLANK RAISES
PAG. 41

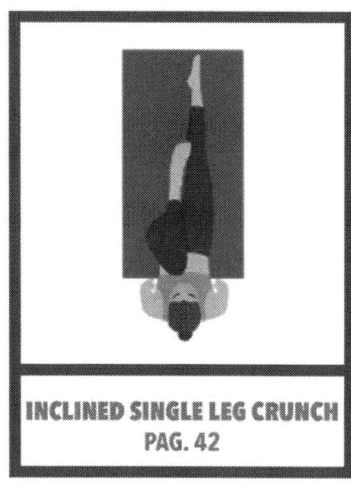

INCLINED SINGLE LEG CRUNCH
PAG. 42

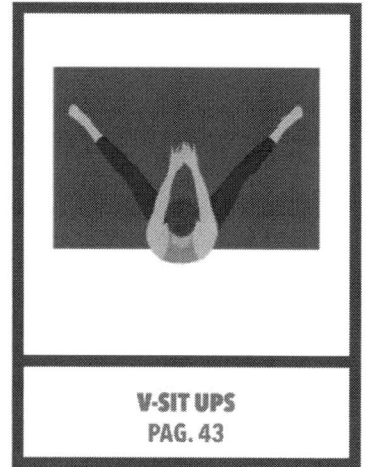

V-SIT UPS
PAG. 43

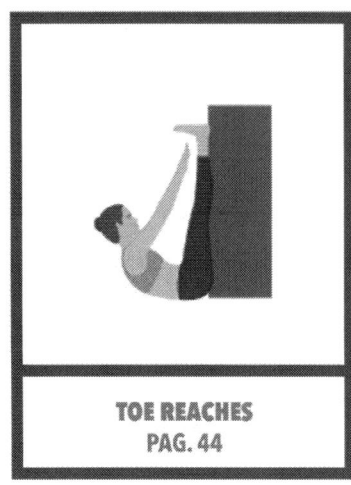

TOE REACHES
PAG. 44

▶▶▶▶ IMPROVING BACK POSTURE - WORKOUTS

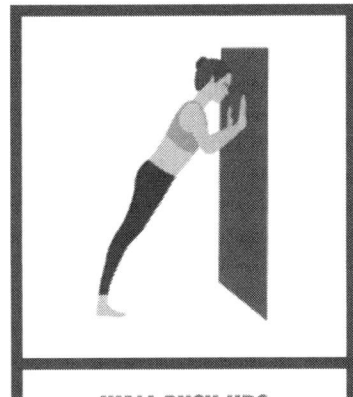

WALL PUSH-UPS
PAG. 46

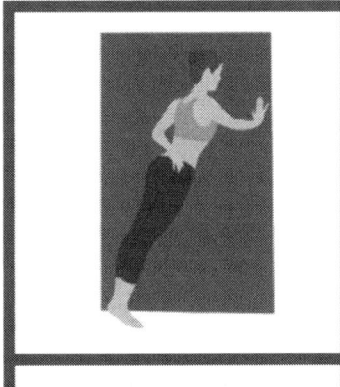

ONE ARM WALL PUSH-UPS
PAG. 47

PLANK SHOULDER TAPS
PAG. 48

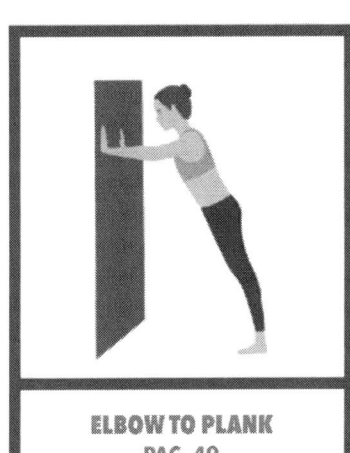

ELBOW TO PLANK
PAG. 49

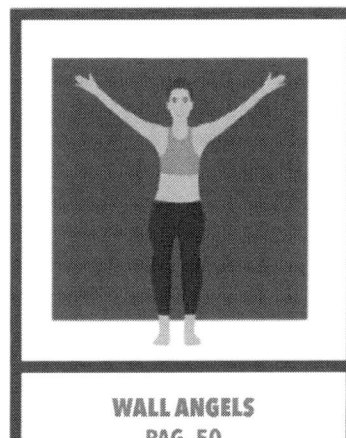

WALL ANGELS
PAG. 50

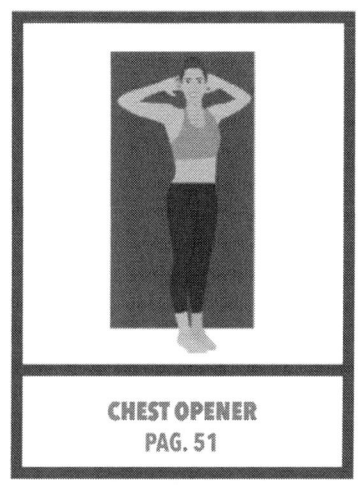

CHEST OPENER
PAG. 51

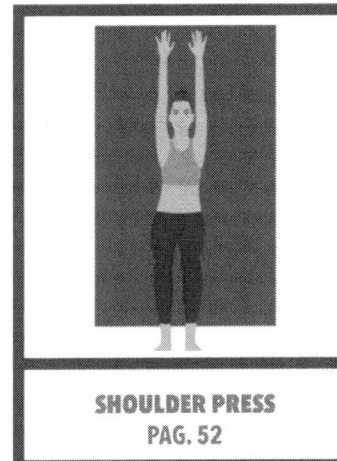

SHOULDER PRESS
PAG. 52

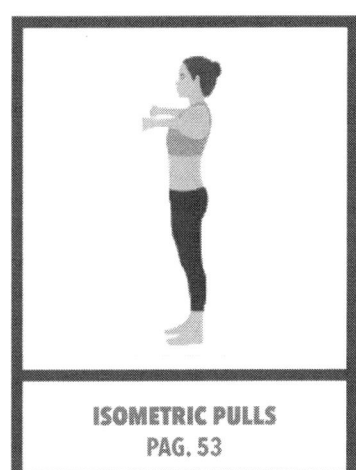

ISOMETRIC PULLS
PAG. 53

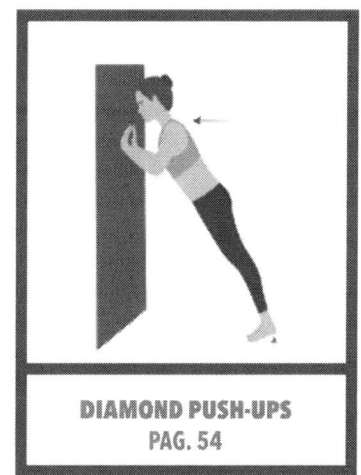

DIAMOND PUSH-UPS
PAG. 54

▶▶▶▶ **IMPROVING BACK POSTURE** - WORKOUTS

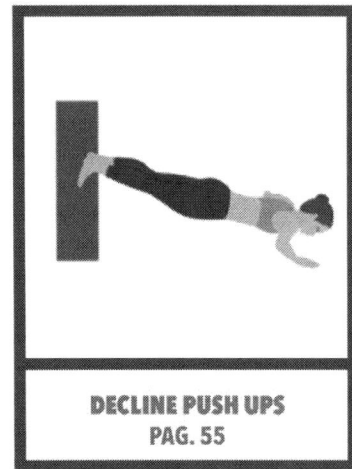
DECLINE PUSH UPS
PAG. 55

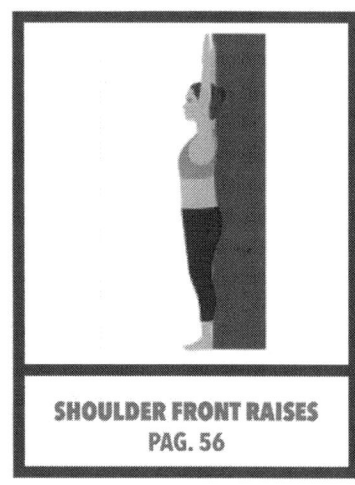
SHOULDER FRONT RAISES
PAG. 56

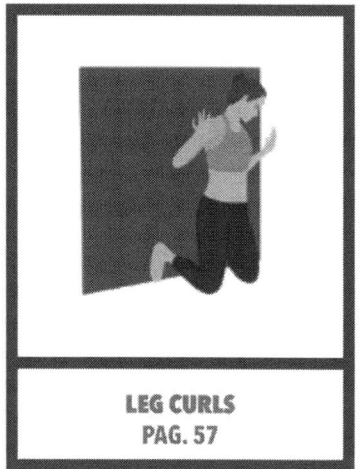
LEG CURLS
PAG. 57

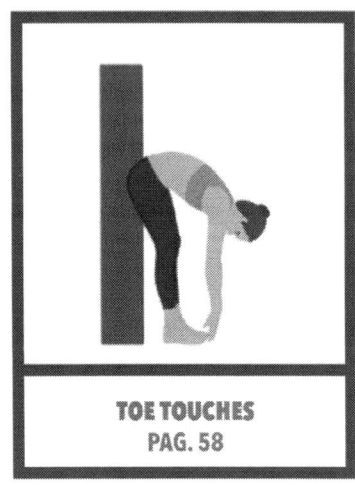
TOE TOUCHES
PAG. 58

▶▶▶▶ SHAPING THE BUTTOCKS - WORKOUTS

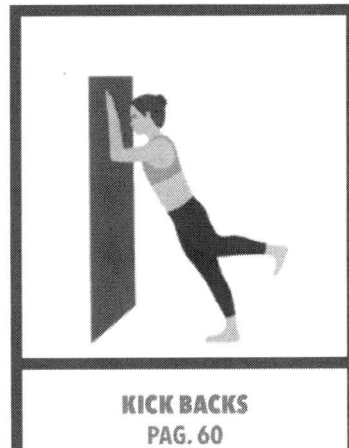
KICK BACKS
PAG. 60

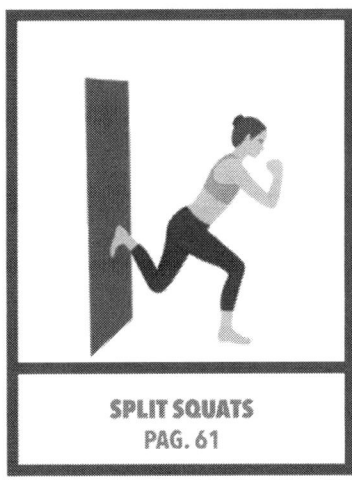
SPLIT SQUATS
PAG. 61

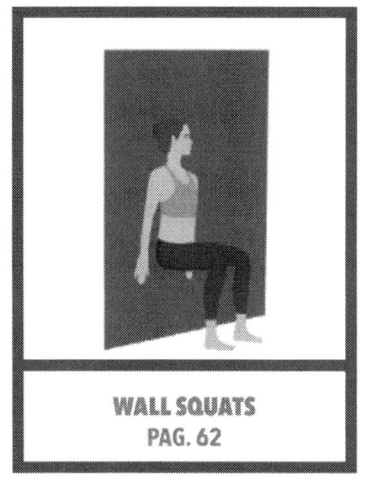
WALL SQUATS
PAG. 62

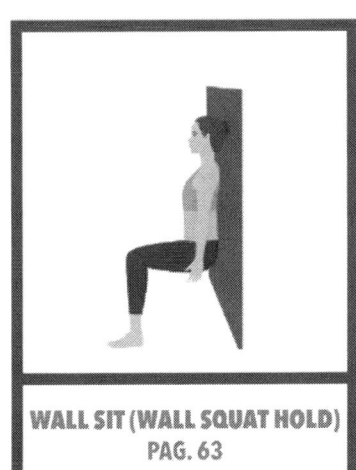
WALL SIT (WALL SQUAT HOLD)
PAG. 63

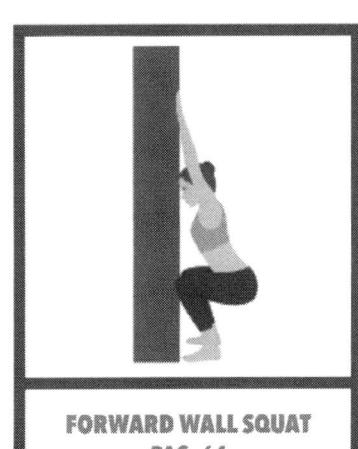
FORWARD WALL SQUAT
PAG. 64

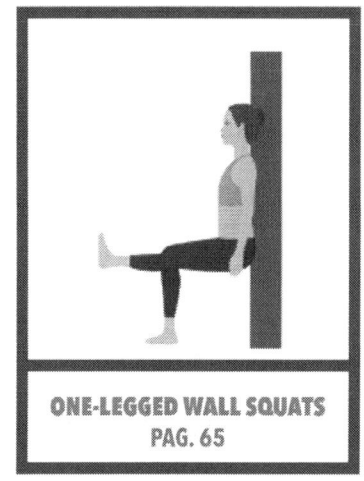
ONE-LEGGED WALL SQUATS
PAG. 65

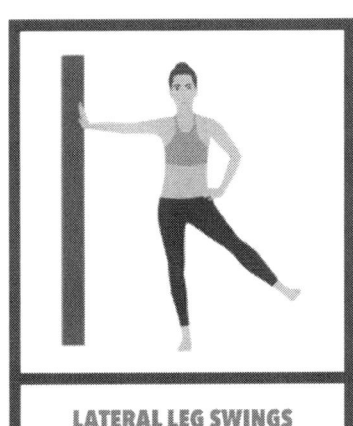
LATERAL LEG SWINGS
PAG. 66

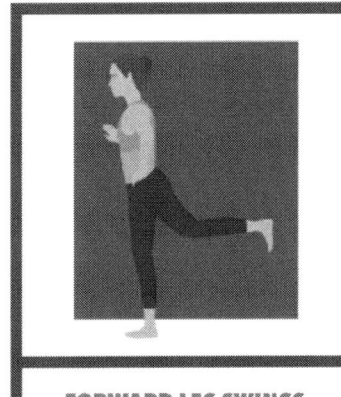
FORWARD LEG SWINGS
PAG. 67

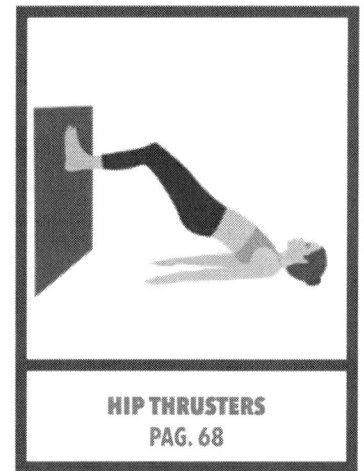
HIP THRUSTERS
PAG. 68

▶▶▶▶ SHAPING THE BUTTOCKS - WORKOUTS

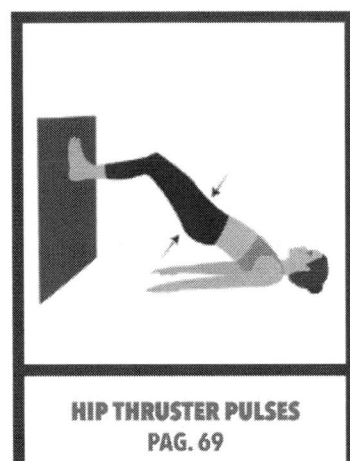
HIP THRUSTER PULSES
PAG. 69

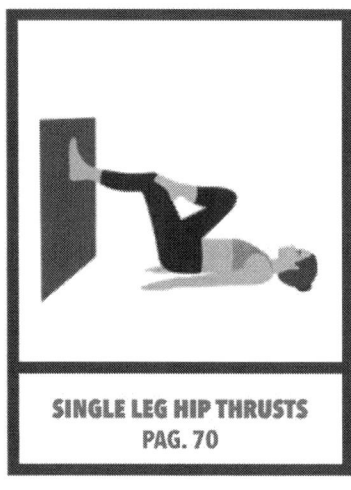
SINGLE LEG HIP THRUSTS
PAG. 70

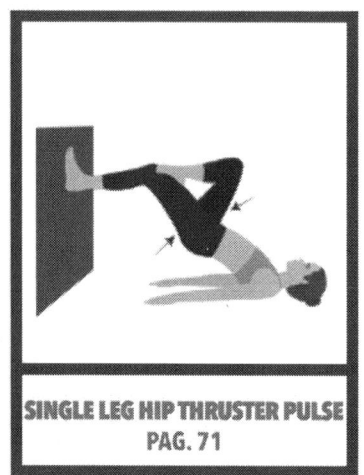
SINGLE LEG HIP THRUSTER PULSE
PAG. 71

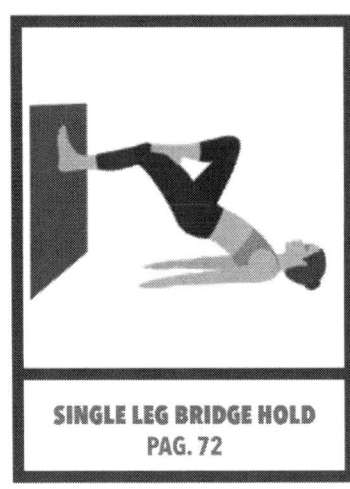
SINGLE LEG BRIDGE HOLD
PAG. 72

INTRODUCTION

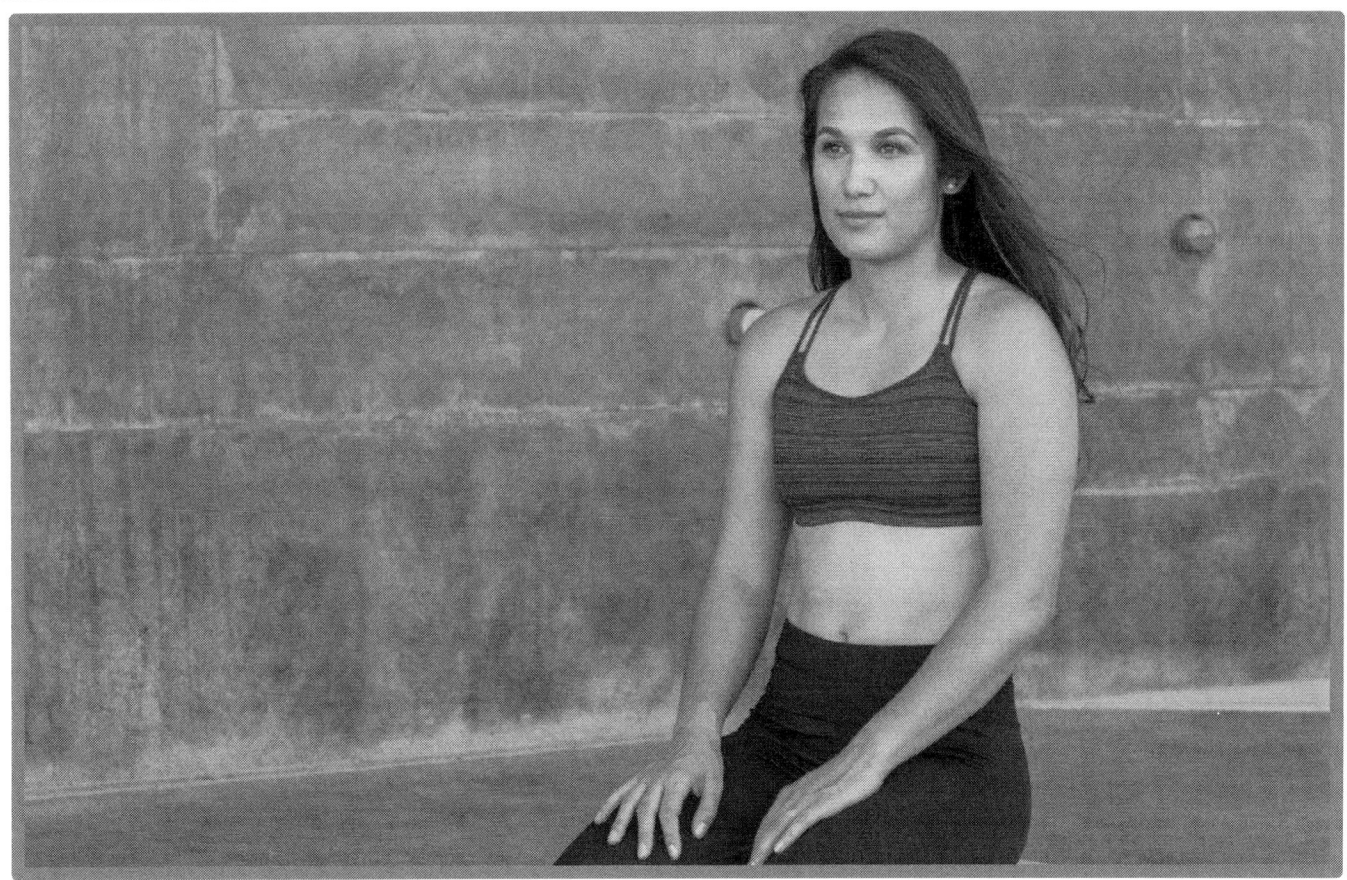

For over a century, Pilates has stood as a testament to the enduring power of mindful exercise. Originally embraced by dancers seeking injury prevention and increased flexibility, this holistic practice has now become a worldwide phenomenon, touching the lives of millions. From Hollywood celebrities to athletes, and even healthcare practitioners, the allure of Pilates is undeniable, often referred to as "having a moment" in the fitness world.

Yet, Pilates is far more than a fleeting trend. Its history is rich and deep-rooted, and a growing body of research supports its myriad physical and mental health benefits. Pilates has been found to enhance core strength and improve flexibility, balance, posture, cognitive function, and overall quality of life.

As the practice evolved over the past century, it incorporated the latest findings in exercise science, rehabilitation, and fitness training. This evolution has made Pilates even more versatile, catering to individuals of all ages, fitness levels, and abilities.

Whether you choose to practice on a mat, utilize specialized equipment, or simply use a wall, Pilates provides a full-body workout accessible to everyone, from beginners to elite athletes.

And, in this book we will delve into the world of Pilates, exploring its roots, its health benefits, and most importantly, how it can be adapted for wall-based exercises. We'll discover how Pilates can transform the way you move and feel, enhancing your overall well-being through mindful movement. So, let's embark on this journey of self-discovery and empowerment, as we explore the unique fusion of Pilates principles and wall-based fitness.

Is Wall Pilates for You?

Pilates, a remarkably adaptable fitness regimen, extends its benefits to a diverse spectrum of individuals. From novices to seasoned fitness enthusiasts, elite athletes, rehabilitation patients, youngsters, seniors, expectant and postpartum mothers, and individuals with physical limitations, Pilates proves to be a versatile exercise system that caters to all.

With a repertoire that boasts thousands of exercise variations and the flexibility to intensify or simplify the challenge, Pilates can be tailored to accommodate the unique needs and capabilities of each practitioner. It offers a safe and efficient workout that can be personalized for everyone.

At its core, Pilates is founded on the principles of biomechanics, delving into the science behind how and why the human body moves as it does. This discipline encompasses the fundamental aspects of motion, force, and momentum. Pilates skillfully applies these principles, allowing for the modification, progression, or regression of exercises using equipment and props to ensure that they remain advantageous for all. Beyond mere mechanics, Pilates incorporates the concept of 'biotensegrity,' emphasizing the synergy between muscular and fascial systems in creating efficient movement (Menzies, 2021).

Pilates takes a holistic approach, targeting overall strength, flexibility, endurance, and body conditioning. It seamlessly complements other forms of exercise, such as cardiovascular workouts, strength training, rehabilitation, or recovery exercises. Athletes, including dancers, golfers, runners, cyclists, and team sports enthusiasts, often incorporate Pilates into their routines to enhance their agility, mobility, and overall performance.

Moreover, Pilates goes beyond physical fitness, promoting mental well-being through its emphasis on mindful breathing, body awareness, and the mind-body connection. Many turn to Pilates for stress relief, during the recovery process from injuries, or chronic pain, or as a preventive measure against future injuries.

A Pilates session isn't just about completing a set number of repetitions; it's about achieving functional movement that aids in daily activities and optimizing the body's efficiency. It's about understanding not just what we do but why we do it. Intention and purpose are integral components of reaching our fitness aspirations.

The Genesis of Pilates: A Brief History

Joseph Pilates, the visionary behind the Pilates method, entered the world in 1883, born to a gymnast father and a naturopath mother in Germany. As a fragile child, he embarked on a journey to enhance his health through physical exercise. His quest led him to delve into various realms of physical fitness, encompassing gymnastics, yoga, boxing, and martial arts.

In a twist of fate, World War I erupted in 1914 while Pilates was in England, engaged in circus performances. He found himself detained and confined in a British prisoner-of-war camp for an extensive four-year period.

During this internment, the foundations of his innovative exercise method began to take shape. Pilates assumed the role of a fitness guide, leading fellow inmates in daily exercise routines and aiding injured soldiers in regaining their strength and mobility through his corrective exercises. One notable anecdote recounts his ingenious idea of attaching springs to hospital beds, allowing bedridden patients to condition their bodies—a concept that later influenced the creation of the renowned Pilates Reformer.

In 1926, Joseph Pilates embarked on a new chapter in the United States. Three years later, alongside his wife Clara, he established a gym in Manhattan, introducing his comprehensive exercise system known as Contrology, which combined mat-based and equipment-assisted exercises. Their studio garnered attention, particularly from the New York dance and performance community, including luminaries such as Martha Graham and George Balanchine. These artists turned to the Pilates method to aid in rehabilitation and injury prevention.

The legacy of Joseph Pilates endured long after his passing in 1967, at the age of 83. Today, Pilates has evolved into a globally recognized fitness method, readily available at boutique studios, franchised fitness centers, community facilities, wellness retreats, and physical therapy clinics across the world.

Reasons Pilates is For You

Before we get on to the book, let us quickly look through a few reasons to strengthen the reason you have picked up the book, to strengthen your whys.

- Enhanced Core Strength: Pilates exercises specifically target a set of crucial muscles including the abdominals, lower back, pelvic floor, and hip muscles. This targeted approach results in improved physical strength and stability, potentially reducing the risk of back pain and pelvic floor issues. These exercises engage deep stabilizers, which are the small muscles that play a pivotal role in supporting and balancing the larger muscle groups.
- Improved Posture and Flexibility: Pilates places a strong emphasis on strengthening the trunk extensor muscles, which in turn promotes optimal alignment of the spine. This focus on the core muscles contributes to better posture. Additionally, Pilates has been shown to enhance flexibility, mobility, balance, and joint range of motion.
- Rehabilitation and Injury Prevention: Pilates has earned recognition as a valuable tool in physical therapy, injury prevention, and rehabilitation. Research indicates its effectiveness in scoliosis and back pain treatment, as well as in preventing injuries among diverse populations, including adults, seniors, and athletes.
- Enhanced Balance and Coordination: Pilates is known to enhance balance and gait performance, particularly in the elderly. By strengthening core muscles and promoting stability, it positively impacts static and dynamic balance. This improvement in balance is not only beneficial for physical health but also contributes to brighter moods and an overall improved quality of life. In fact, it is often incorporated into fall prevention programs to boost balance capabilities.
- Stress and Anxiety Reduction: The mindful aspects of Pilates, including intentional breathing, body awareness, and mindfulness, have demonstrated effectiveness in stress and anxiety management. These practices are associated with reduced cortisol levels, providing a calming effect on the mind and body.
- Sports Performance Enhancement: Pilates is increasingly recommended as cross-training for athletes across various sports disciplines. Its emphasis on balance, agility, flexibility, mobility, and the strengthening of deep stabilizing muscles around joints and the torso makes it a valuable addition to training regimens. Pilates has been shown to positively impact sports performance and reduce the risk of injuries.

Now that we have gained a comprehensive understanding of the fundamental principles of Pilates, it's time to embark on an exploration of the intriguing world of Wall Pilates. In the upcoming chapters, we will delve deeper into the essence of Wall Pilates, uncover its unique attributes, and discover how it can further elevate our physical and mental well-being. Get ready to immerse yourself in the transformative journey that Wall Pilates has to offer.

CHAPTER 1. WHY WALL PILATES

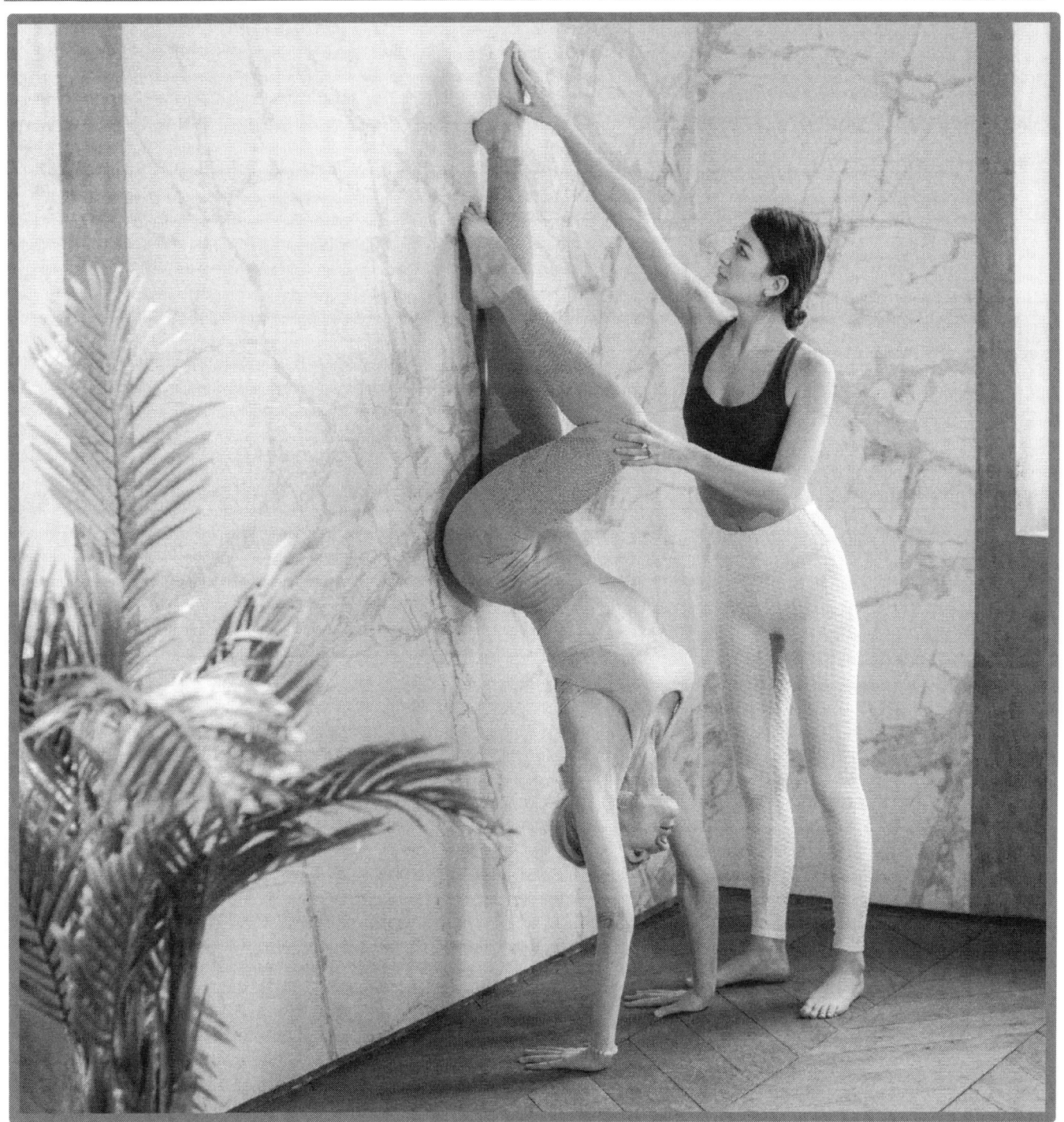

If you are already a fan of Pilates and you are looking for a refreshing twist on your workout routine, then you ought to dive into the world of Wall Pilates. If you are not a fan, wall Pilates will, for sure, turn you into one for this is a fabulous fusion of fitness and fun that will have you hooked from the very first move.

Joseph Pilates, the genius behind the original Pilates method pioneered this revolutionary concept by using walls and props to help his clients perfect their form and alignment. Today, passionate instructors have taken his innovative ideas and transformed them into the vibrant fitness phenomenon known as Wall Pilates.

So, what's the buzz all about? Wall Pilates is like the glamorous cousin of traditional Pilates, bringing a whole new dimension to core strengthening. Instead of relying solely on body weight and gravity, we're turning up the resistance dial by incorporating the power of the wall. The result? Toned abs, sculpted arms, and a fabulous booty that won't quit, all wrapped up in one accessible workout.

Whether you're just starting your fitness journey or you're a seasoned pro looking to push your limits, Wall Pilates has something special for you. This versatile workout caters to all levels and tastes, making it a must-try for every fitness enthusiast.

Now, if you've dabbled in Pilates before, you're probably familiar with classics like glute bridges and the iconic hundred. Well, picture this: You replace the ball, band, or reformer machine with a trusty wall. Voila, you're officially a Wall Pilates enthusiast! Translation: Wall Pilates is a creative twist on mat Pilates, where you'll press body parts, mainly your feet, against the wall while performing exercises like the hundred, wall squats, or planks. The wall isn't just for support; it's your secret weapon, adding that extra resistance to amplify the burn.

While your glutes and core will definitely feel the love in Wall Pilates, don't worry, your upper body won't be left out of the action. We're talking about standing exercises that target your arms and chest, like wall push-ups and planks. It's a full-body experience that will leave you feeling strong, confident, and utterly fabulous.

But what makes Pilates, in any form, so remarkable? It's not just about physical strength; it's a low-impact workout that nourishes both body and mind. Pilates blends six key principles: concentration, control, centering, flow, precision, and breathing. These principles guide you through precise, controlled, and purposeful movements, all while sharpening your focus and enhancing body awareness.

Wall Pilates is the evolution of mat Pilates that you can rock right in the comfort of your own home, using nothing more than a trusty wall. It's a fantastic way to spice up your workouts and infuse a dash of flavor into traditional Pilates moves.

And why do we choose the wall as our workout BFF? Simple. It provides the support and stability you need as you stretch and sculpt your muscles, all while adding that extra challenge to keep things exciting.

So, girl, if you're ready to embark on a fitness journey that's both empowering and exhilarating, Wall Pilates is your ticket to a stronger, more confident you. Let's embrace the wall and unleash the power within!

Benefits of Pilates

Have you ever wondered about the science behind the Pilates craze and the incredible benefits it offers? Well, let's dive into a fascinating paper by June Kloubec, published in the scientific journal Muscles Ligaments Tendons J. in 2011, which sheds light on the many advantages of Pilates:

- Transversus Abdominis: First things first, let's talk about our lower abdominal superhero, the transversus abdominis. This muscle, located just below the belly button, plays a pivotal role in Pilates. Before every Pilates move, we're cued to engage it by simply "pulling in" the lower abdomen. Why is this so important? Well, this muscle is a champion of posture control. It's the very first muscle to kick into action when we make any limb movement. Think of it as your secret weapon for maintaining trunk stability during dynamic motions.
- Breathing Matters: Pilates isn't just about movement; it's also about mastering the art of breathing. Proper breathing techniques are essential to generate sufficient intra-abdominal pressure, which in turn aids in stabilizing our lower back. Plus, learning to breathe right reduces the sensation of fatigue and effort during exercise, making your Pilates journey a breeze.
- Abdominal Exercises: Pilates gives us a wide array of abdominal exercises to challenge and strengthen our core muscles. Unlike some traditional exercises that might not provide enough muscle activation, Pilates steps up the game. It's all about achieving a balance between challenging those abdominal muscles while keeping the load on the lower back minimal, which is particularly vital for our overall well-being.
- Body Position and Posture: This form of exercise emphasizes specific body positions and posture. It encourages a slight forward flexion of the neck, scapula stabilization, and connecting the rib cage to the hips. These adjustments optimize spinal alignment and muscle engagement. It's like setting the stage for your body to perform at its best and achieve maximum muscle contraction.
- Low Back Pain (LBP): One of the most significant areas where Pilates shines is in the treatment of low back pain. Core weakness is a common issue associated with LBP, and Pilates is all about strengthening the core. It integrates stabilization and axial elongation into every exercise, helping you avoid undue stress on your back. Studies have shown that Pilates-based approaches are effective in reducing pain and disability in individuals with chronic low back pain.
- Additional Uses: Pilates isn't just limited to back pain relief; it has a wide range of applications. It's been explored for postoperative rehabilitation, fall prevention in the elderly, pelvic floor

strengthening, and even weight management. Research indicates its potential benefits in these areas, showing improved functional capacity, posture, and quality of life.

Apart from the scientific proofs, the following are the overall benefits that are empirical, that I have experienced with my practice. In our modern, often sedentary lives, we spend prolonged hours sitting at desks, which can lead to discomfort, especially in the back. Weak core muscles and poor posture can exacerbate this problem. Wall Pilates comes to the rescue by offering an effective solution. When we talk about core strength, it's not just the abdominal muscles; it includes the muscles in your back and sides as well. Wall Pilates provides the stability your spine needs, enabling you to concentrate on engaging those deep abdominal muscles effectively, which can sometimes be challenging with mat Pilates alone. The wall becomes your ally in fostering better posture and enhancing core strength, an essential aspect of overall fitness.

Muscular endurance is the ability of your muscles to sustain contractions against resistance for an extended duration, a vital component of functional fitness. It's what allows you to perform everyday activities with ease, like carrying groceries or lifting your little ones. Wall Pilates contributes significantly to improving both muscular strength and endurance. It achieves this through deliberate, controlled movement patterns and by extending the "time under tension," an important concept in progressive overload. The wall's presence also adds extra resistance, effectively enabling you to incorporate a "weight-like" challenge into your exercises without requiring actual weights.

While I'm a firm advocate of weightlifting, the flexibility aspect often takes a backseat. You might find that despite being able to deadlift a substantial load, touching your toes remains a challenge. Wall Pilates, known for its capacity to enhance flexibility while building muscle, can help bridge this gap. What's particularly beneficial is that the wall can be ingeniously integrated into stretches, facilitating deeper stretches and expanding your range of motion. This flexibility is invaluable for various exercises and daily movements.

Consider the force exerted on your joints during physical activities as their "impact." High-impact exercises, such as running and jumping, can place significant stress on your joints and feet, potentially causing discomfort, especially for those new to exercise or recovering from injuries. In contrast, low-impact exercises, like walking and stepping, reduce strain on your joints. Wall Pilates belongs to this category, making it an excellent choice for individuals dealing with joint pain or recovering from injuries that restrict mobility. It's frequently incorporated into rehabilitation programs due to its low-impact nature, offering the dual benefits of strengthening the core, enhancing flexibility, and improving muscular endurance. The wall can serve as a supportive companion for those on the path to recovery or as a tool for easing into more challenging positions, all while prioritizing joint health and comfort.

So, Pilates is not just a trendy fad or a fashion statement; it's backed by science and offers a plethora of benefits. Whether you're looking to strengthen your core, alleviate back pain, improve posture, or enhance your overall well-being, Pilates has got you covered. It's a versatile and empowering fitness method that can benefit women of all ages and fitness levels. So why wait? But why dive into the world of Pilates and unlock your inner strength and grace, when there are options such as yoga and HIIT? The next section of this chapter deals exactly with this question.

Yoga vs. Pilates:
Unveiling the Differences and Common Ground

In the realm of low-impact exercises, two practices, Yoga and Pilates, often take center stage. They share the attribute of being gentle on the body while bestowing a multitude of physical and mental benefits. However, they diverge in their approach, making them distinct paths to holistic wellness.

Yoga: A Spiritual Fusion of Postures and Mindfulness

Yoga, originating in ancient India, marries physical poses, known as asanas, with breath control techniques called pranayama. It is, at its core, a holistic practice, often referred to as meditative movement. The beauty of yoga lies in its versatility, with various styles catering to different needs and abilities.

Pilates: Core-Centric Strength and Precision

On the other hand, Pilates is a discipline that places a premium on core strength and precision. Joseph Pilates, a man who developed this practice, devised it as a way to enhance muscular strength, flexibility, and overall body control. While yoga encompasses a wide array of poses and flow sequences, Pilates embraces small, controlled movements that zero in on specific muscle groups.

Strength and Flexibility: The Shared Goals

Both Yoga and Pilates share the common objectives of enhancing strength and flexibility. Yoga, through its diverse postures and flows, encourages the stretching and strengthening of muscles. Meanwhile, Pilates adopts a disciplined approach, emphasizing core strength as the foundational pillar. It not only targets the core but also extends its benefits to muscle toning, overall strength, and body control.

Mindfulness and Stress Relief: A Mental Oasis

The mental benefits of Yoga and Pilates extend far beyond physical wellness. Both practices foster mindfulness and stress relief, offering solace in our busy lives. Yoga, as a holistic system, is as much about nurturing the mind and spirit as it is about physical postures. It encourages meditation, connecting with the body, breath, and mind—an opportunity to slow down and introspect.

Pilates, while not delving into meditation like Yoga, engages the mind through concentration on body movements and breath control. It creates a meditative and stress-relieving space, allowing practitioners to find balance in the present moment.

Rehabilitation and Injury Prevention: Tailored Approaches

For those on the path to recovery or seeking injury prevention, both Yoga and Pilates hold value. Pilates, with its slow, controlled movements, proves beneficial for rehabilitation. It offers adaptable solutions for individuals dealing with injuries or chronic pain, promoting restorative effects, especially for lower back pain and poor posture.

Yoga, known for its deep stretches and flexibility-enhancing postures, aids in preventing sports injuries and alleviating muscle tension. Its diverse styles cater to various needs, making it a valuable tool for athletes and fitness enthusiasts alike.

The Choice: Personal Preferences and Goals

In the eternal debate of Yoga versus Pilates, there's no definitive winner. The choice ultimately hinges on personal preferences and wellness goals. If your aim is to fortify your core, enhance precision, and indulge in a structured, low-impact workout, Pilates may be your calling. On the other hand, if you seek an all-encompassing approach to wellness, fostering strength, flexibility, and mindfulness, Yoga might be your path to holistic health.

So, ladies, whether you find solace in the serenity of Yoga or the precision of Pilates, remember that both these practices share a common thread—they are your companions on the journey to a healthier, more balanced you. Though this book focuses on Pilates, I would embrace the one that resonates with your heart and soul, and relish the manifold rewards of a nourished body and mind. But, if you are able to embrace both these disciplines, you for sure are going to benefit from both, especially because, as we can see, they complement each other.

HIIT vs. Pilates:
Unpacking the Contrasts and Synergies

In the realm of fitness, HIIT (High-Intensity Interval Training) and Pilates emerge as two prominent contenders, each offering a distinct approach to achieving health and fitness goals. These two methods stand apart in their philosophy, yet they share common ground when it comes to contributing to overall well-being.

HIIT: Intense Efficiency for Cardiovascular Fitness

HIIT, an abbreviation for High-Intensity Interval Training, is a newcomer known for its efficiency. It thrives on the principle of delivering maximum results in minimal time. HIIT workouts involve short, vigorous bursts of exercise, or intervals, interspersed with brief rest periods. These intervals must elevate the heart rate to around 80% of its maximum capacity to qualify as true HIIT workouts.

Pilates: Deliberate Precision and Mindful Movement

In contrast, Pilates offers a serene counterpoint to the intensity of HIIT. A typical Pilates session extends between 45 minutes to an hour, focusing on slow, deliberate movements that aim to strengthen the body, improve posture, and enhance flexibility. Pilates embodies a mindful practice more than a workout, emphasizing precision and deep engagement of muscles.

Divergent Goals and Fitness Focus

The choice between HIIT and Pilates hinges on your fitness goals and preferences. HIIT is tailored for those who prioritize cardiovascular endurance and fat burning. It offers a structured approach to shedding pounds, boosting aerobic capacity, and targeting specific areas. On the other hand, Pilates champions strength development, flexibility, and a deliberate, unhurried journey toward physical and mental well-being.

A Blend of Forces: The Power of Integration

Rather than a competition, experts advocate for a harmonious blend of both HIIT and Pilates in one's fitness routine. The rationale lies in the fact that our bodies operate through two distinct energy systems—one activated during low-intensity training like Pilates and another engaged in high-intensity endeavors like HIIT.

The fusion of these two approaches ensures comprehensive fitness. HIIT excels in torching calories, invigorating metabolism, and enhancing cardiovascular health. Meanwhile, Pilates offers core stability, muscle strength, and mindfulness. By integrating both, you access the holistic benefits of exercise, nurturing your body's diverse needs.

Recovery and Injury Prevention: Pilates as a Companion

While HIIT can be a potent calorie burner, its high-impact nature raises injury concerns, particularly when form and technique aren't carefully observed. For those engaged in HIIT and recovering from injuries,

Pilates becomes an invaluable ally. Pilates aids in rehabilitation and injury prevention by reinforcing the core, promoting body awareness, and ensuring proper alignment.

Mind and Body Harmony: Stress Reduction with Pilates

Stress, whether mental or physical, can take a toll on the body. HIIT workouts, while effective, can exacerbate stress if overdone. In contrast, Pilates provides a meditative experience, fusing body awareness with breath control. This mindful aspect fosters relaxation, reduces cortisol levels, and bolsters overall well-being.

Joint Health and Longevity: Pilates' Gentle Embrace

Lastly, preserving joint health is a paramount concern. HIIT, with its high-impact movements, can place undue stress on joints. Pilates, being low-impact, offers a gentler alternative. It not only supports joint longevity but also serves as an excellent foundation for those venturing into more intense training methods, mitigating the risk of overexertion.

In the ongoing HIIT vs. Pilates debate, the ultimate winner emerges as the harmonious coexistence of both. By leveraging their respective strengths and addressing unique fitness needs, individuals can craft a balanced fitness regimen that reaps the rewards of strength, endurance, flexibility, and mindfulness–a holistic approach to lifelong health and well-being.

Now, What Should You Choose?

Taking on Wall Pilates is an immersive venture into holistic well-being, where numerous facets of health and vitality converge. At its core, Pilates radiates strength, and not just in the muscular sense. This practice fortifies the body's epicenter, the core, cultivating resilience that ripples outward to transform your life.

Beyond the surface, Pilates becomes a powerful conduit for change. It is an elixir for posture, transcending slouching and discomfort, ushering in an era of effortless alignment and vitality. Back pain, once a relentless companion, finds solace in the nurturing embrace of Pilates.

But Pilates is not confined to the realms of physicality; it extends a compassionate hand to your emotional well-being. Stress, that silent assailant, finds its foe in the inward focus and breath mastery of Pilates. As you journey deeper within, a newfound awareness of self and surroundings emerges, casting a soothing spell on frazzled nerves.

Furthermore, Pilates is not just a solo endeavor; it embraces diverse aspects of your life. It champions balance, fostering an equilibrium that harmonizes your movements and transcends into everyday activities. A resilient immune system stands as a testament to Pilates' ability to elevate health.

Yet, Pilates does not stop at the borders of your body; it extends to your mind. Cognitive faculties flourish, with markers of improved neuron development, enhanced blood flow to the brain, and longevity of memory. This mental vitality finds a companion in motivation, igniting an intrinsic drive to persist and thrive.

And in the most intimate of spaces, Pilates enhances your life's pleasures. Its influence extends to the bedroom, where it not only fosters endurance but also strengthens the pelvic floor, heightening sensations of pleasure.

Ultimately, Pilates is the conductor of a symphony of wellness. It amplifies sports performance, promotes bone density, and ignites a radiant mood. Sleep, that elusive treasure, becomes more attainable, and a sense of play infuses your fitness journey with joy.

In essence, Pilates isn't just an exercise routine; it's a transformational odyssey that transcends the boundaries of physicality, nurturing your body, mind, and spirit. It's an investment in your holistic well-being, where strength, balance, and vitality converge, illuminating the path to a more vibrant and enriched life.

In Conclusion,

Wall Pilates, at its core, is not just a strength exercise in the muscular sense. The practice not only fortifies the body's core, it also helps us work on our mental fortitude. It works on our posture, and helps get rid of slouching and back pain. The exercise, as mentioned above, is not purely confined to the realms of physicality; it extends a compassionate hand to our emotional well-being, helping to rid ourselves of stress, through inward focus and the mastery of breath.

And as you begin to explore the limitations and extents of your body movements, a newfound awareness of self and surroundings emerges. It is also shown to contribute to a stronger immune system, boosting the body's defense mechanisms. While it's not a replacement for a healthy lifestyle and proper nutrition, it certainly plays a role in overall well-being.

When your overall-being improves, an elevation in cognitive function is the automatic result. The enhanced blood flow to the brain helps with focus, memory, and overall mental clarity. Moreover, the mental aspect of Pilates, which emphasizes concentration and precision, can be a great way to unwind while improving executive functioning skills. And all this, like a chain reaction, can ignite an internal motivation to stick with your fitness routine. The sense of achievement that comes with mastering different movements and pushing your body to its limits can be a powerful motivator to persist and thrive in your overall wellness journey.

What's more, Pilates is shown to have a positive impact on your intimate life. It can help improve endurance and strengthen the pelvic floor muscles, which can lead to heightened sensations of pleasure and a more satisfying intimate life.

Most importantly, incorporating Pilates into your routine can infuse a sense of play and joy into your fitness journey. It's not just a workout; it's an opportunity to explore and enjoy the movements of your body.

CHAPTER 2. BEFORE YOU START

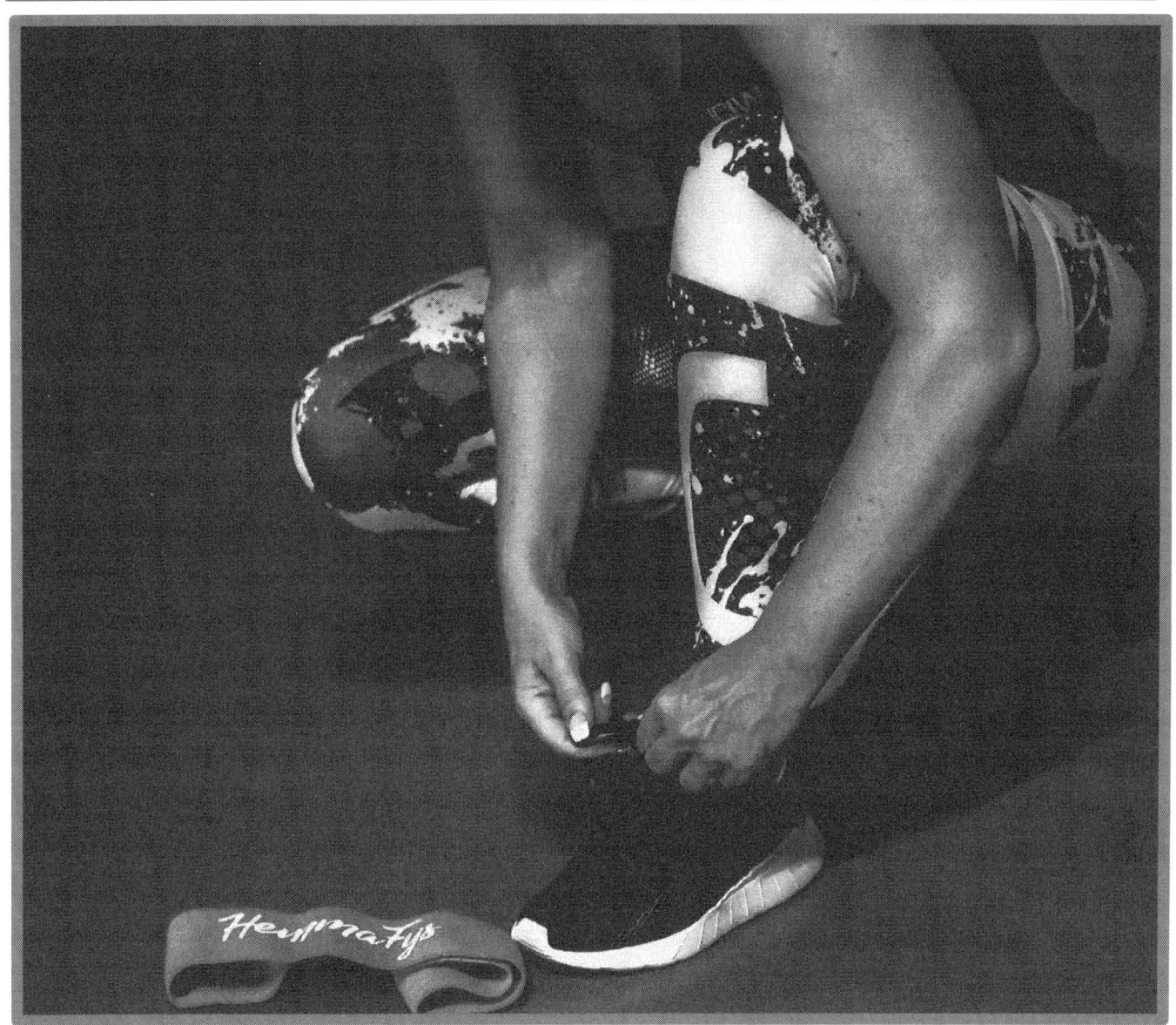

Within the pages of this book, we delve deeply into the realm of wall exercises and their scientifically proven impact on the body. Our exploration primarily centers on key areas of the physique, namely the abdominal muscles, the back, posture, and the gluteal region. What truly distinguishes this book is its remarkable flexibility, granting you, the reader, the freedom to choose your desired focus.

If you're eager to cultivate robust abdominal strength, flip to chapter 3, where we delve into the transformative world of wall Pilates exercises designed to chisel and tone your core. Alternatively, if you seek relief from back discomfort and yearn for a healthier spine, Chapter 4 provides a tailored approach to fortify your back muscles and enhance your overall well-being.

For those who aspire to exude confidence through impeccable posture, Chapter 5 offers an in-depth exploration of posture-improving wall exercises that will have you standing tall and feeling more self-assured.

And let's not forget the allure of sculpting those glutes into their best shape ever. Whichever area you choose to focus on, rest assured that this book empowers you to embark on a personalized wall Pilates journey, putting you in control of your fitness destiny. So, go ahead and take charge of your exercise routine with the knowledge and flexibility provided within these pages.

A List of All You Need

In terms of equipment, what you don't need with wall pilates is a list. This exercise routine not only adds an intriguing twist to essential exercises by seamlessly integrating the wall for added support, but it also is simple to get started on. Carve out just 20 to 45 minutes of your daily schedule to embark on this engaging practice. You have the option to structure your session by completing each exercise in multiple sets or going through the entire circuit three times, with brief one-minute interludes in between. Precision and control are your guiding principles throughout this workout, necessitating unwavering core engagement.

For optimal stability and safety, we recommend performing these exercises without footwear, reducing the risk of any unexpected slips or discomfort. However, do ensure your feet are clean, as we wouldn't want any marks on your pristine walls. Also, don't forget to get yourself a yoga mat, for it not only serves as a cushioning buffer for your joints, shielding them from the harsh impact of a solid floor but also boasts a non-slip texture that ensures you remain securely anchored, even during those challenging and contorted positions. Embark on this transformative journey, where the wall becomes your trusted partner, elevating your Wall Pilates experience and sculpting your physique with finesse.

Your Mindset

Initiating this fitness journey can be particularly challenging due to the mental aspect. While the equipment requirements are minimal and the workouts are accommodating for individuals of various sizes, convincing the mind to engage in beneficial and healthy activities can be a formidable task. Here are several valuable tips to help you kickstart your journey:

Embrace Social Fitness

Motivating yourself to exercise can be a challenging task, even when you genuinely enjoy the activity. A great way to kickstart your wall pilates journey is by involving friends or family. Share your fitness goals with them and work together to hold each other accountable. For many, exercise becomes an opportunity to bond with loved ones. Consider establishing a weekly hiking routine with your family or joining a city-league sports team with a friend. Remember, the more, the merrier!

Be Patient With Yourself

When you embarked on your journey to learn painting, did you master every brushstroke on day one? Certainly not. Learning a new skill takes time and patience. Your motivation and skill level will have their ups and downs, and you might encounter setbacks that require you to take a break. Don't be too hard on yourself if developing a passion for exercise doesn't happen as quickly as you'd like. Cultivating a new enthusiasm doesn't always happen overnight.

Explore New Horizons, Then Keep Exploring

We all have that one friend who absolutely adores running. Running makes them feel alive and exhilarated. However, for many of us, lacing up our running shoes feels more like a chore than a joy. Remember, not everyone will derive the same pleasure from the same sport or activity. Be open to experimenting and finding joy in the world of fitness. Think outside the box–try cross-country skiing, enroll in a boxing class, engage in a friendly soccer match with your kids, participate in a dog agility class, or even pick up a pair of rollerblades. There's no limit to the number of sports you can explore. When you find the right fit (or fits!) for you, it will click, just as it did for your running enthusiast friend.

Relish Rest Days Without Guilt

Overexertion can quickly lead to burnout and demotivation. Even if you've discovered a form of exercise that you truly enjoy, it's essential to incorporate rest days into your routine. These days of rest give your body the chance to recover and help reduce the risk of injury. So, savor your well-deserved rest days! It's perfectly okay to unwind on the couch, enjoy a bit of extra sleep, or indulge in a binge-watching session of your favorite TV series. You've earned those rest days, and they are an integral part of your fitness journey.

Discover Your "Why"

This is perhaps the most crucial element of your fitness journey–it works best when the motivation comes from purpose. External sources of motivation, such as encouragement from loved ones or medical professionals, may not always suffice, it has to come from within and the best way it can come from within is by fabricating a purpose around the activity. It's essential to make your fitness journey personal and find your own driving force.

Your "why" can be anything—from weight loss and competition to a genuine love for the sport, stress reduction, or quality time with your children. Your "why" is the powerful force that will propel you out of bed and into your workout gear.

CHAPTER 3. ACHIEVING TONE ABS

How does Wall Pilates benefit your abdominal muscles? Wall Pilates employs the support of a wall to facilitate a comprehensive workout that not only engages your abdominal muscles but also targets your back muscles. When it comes to strengthening your abs, here's how it operates:

- Enhancing Core Strength and Posture: Wall Pilates prioritizes core muscle strengthening, aiding in the maintenance of a healthy posture while safeguarding your spinal health.
- Boosting Abdominal Strength and Stability: Through regular practice, you can develop increased abdominal strength and stability, enabling you to execute more advanced exercises with confidence.
- Efficient Muscle Engagement: By involving multiple muscle groups simultaneously, Wall Pilates proves to be a highly efficient approach for achieving well-defined abs quickly.
- Improving Posture: This practice contributes to improved posture, eliminating the slouched posture that can obscure the definition of your abdominal muscles.

Here are some valuable pointers to maximize the effectiveness of your Wall Pilates routine for lower abs:

- Maintain Correct Form and Alignment: Ensure your body maintains proper alignment during Wall Pilates exercises for your abs. This precaution guarantees that you engage the right muscle groups while minimizing the risk of strain on your spine or other body areas.
- Mindful Breathing: Focus on slow, deep breaths as you engage in Wall Pilates exercises. This deliberate breathing technique enhances your concentration and optimizes the benefits of your workout.
- Gradual Progression: Avoid attempting high-intensity Wall Pilates routines right from the start. Instead, commence with a lower intensity level and progressively increase your repetitions as your strength improves.

By incorporating these mindset-oriented approaches, you can harness the full potential of Wall Pilates for your abdominal muscles.

Workouts

▶▷▶▷ BRIDGE RAISES

Target: Glutes, hamstrings, and core muscles
Number of sets: 3
Repetitions per set: 10 to 15 reps

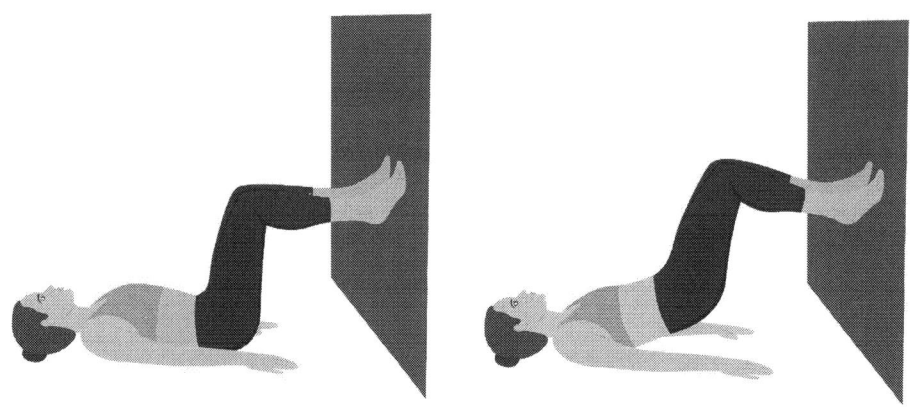

Steps

1. Lay flat on your back–feel free to use an exercise mat. Place your feet close to the wall.
2. Bend your knees at a 90-degree angle, and rest your arms comfortably at your sides.
3. Engage your core muscles by sucking your belly button toward your spine. This will provide stability during the movement.
4. Gently press your feet against the wall, using it as leverage.
5. As you exhale, slowly lift your hips off the mat, pushing them upward toward the ceiling.
6. Continue raising your hips until your body is in a straight line from your shoulders to your knees.
7. At the top of the bridge, pause for a moment, ensuring your glutes and core muscles are engaged.
8. Keep your weight evenly distributed between your feet and shoulders.
9. Inhale as you begin to lower your hips back down to the mat, one vertebra at a time.
10. Ensure a controlled descent, maintaining the engagement of your core and buttock muscles throughout.
11. Rest briefly between sets.

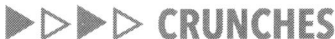 **CRUNCHES**

Target: Abs, and core muscles
Number of sets: 3
Repetitions per set: 10 to 15 reps

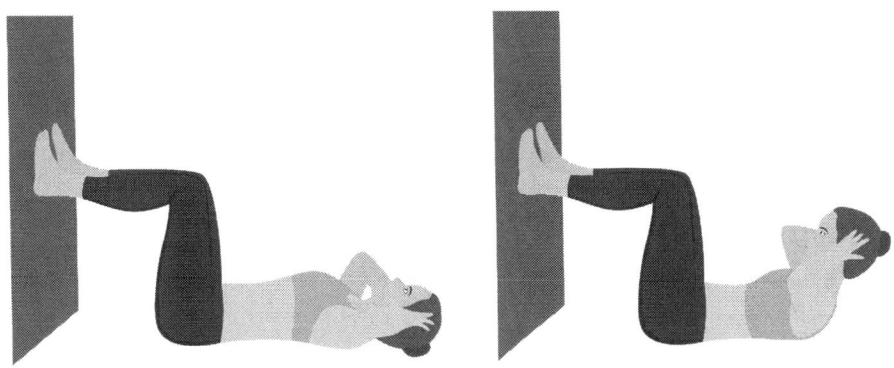

Steps

1. Lie down on your back and extend your legs vertically, pressing your feet against the wall.
2. Place your hands lightly on the sides of your head, with your elbows pointing out to the sides.
3. Engage your core by sucking your belly button in toward your spine. This will help maintain stability during the movement.
4. Exhale as you lift your head, neck, and shoulders off the mat. Focus on engaging your abdominal muscles when performing the crunch.
5. Simultaneously, bring your chest closer to your knees, keeping your lower back on the mat.
6. Ensure your chin is slightly tucked to avoid straining your neck and maintain a smooth, controlled movement.
7. At the peak of the crunch, briefly hold the position and contract your abdominal muscles.
8. Feel the tension in your core before beginning to lower your upper body back down.
9. Inhale as you slowly lower your head, neck, and shoulders back to the mat.
10. Maintain core engagement throughout the lowering phase.

▶▷▶▷ CRUNCH TWISTER

Target: Abs, and core muscles
Number of sets: 3
Repetitions per set: 20 to 30 reps (10 to 15 reps per side)

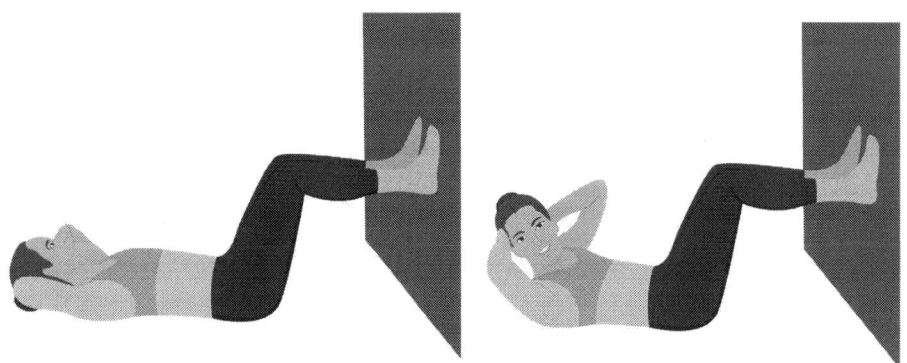

Steps

1. Begin by positioning yourself on an exercise mat with your back to the wall.
2. Lie down on your back and extend your legs at 90 degrees. Press your feet against the wall.
3. Place your hands lightly behind your head, with your elbows pointing out to the sides.
4. Engage your core by sucking your belly button in toward your spine. This will help maintain stability during the movement.
5. Exhale as you lift your head, neck, and shoulders off the mat, similar to the starting position for crunches.
6. As you crunch upward, simultaneously bring your right elbow toward your left knee, aiming to make contact between them (get as close as you possibly can).
7. Lower your upper body back down, but keep your head slightly raised off the mat.
8. Inhale as you lower your head back to the mat.
9. As you exhale, lift your head, neck, and shoulders again, but this time bring your left elbow toward your right knee.
10. Lower your upper body back down.
11. Alternate between bringing your right elbow to your left knee and your left elbow to your right knee.
12. Maintain a controlled pace throughout the exercise.
13. Rest briefly between sets, and aim to perform a total of three sets.

▶▷▶▷ BRIDGE KNEE TO CHEST EXERCISE

Target: Abs and core muscles
Number of sets: 3
Repetitions per set: 20 to 30 reps (10 to 15 reps per side)

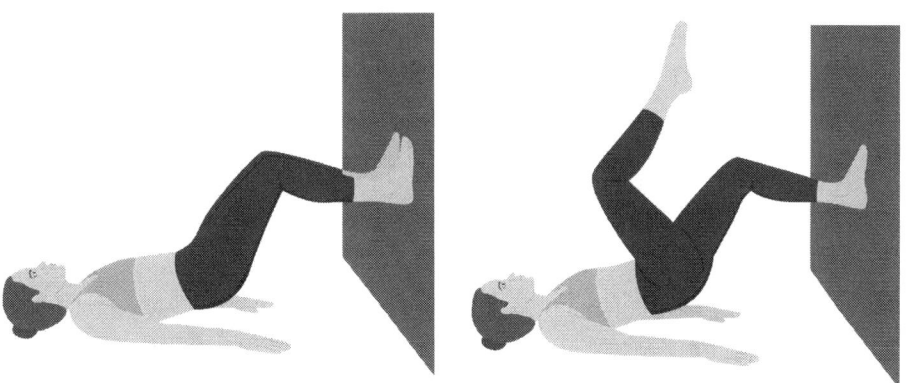

Steps

1. Start by lying on your back on an exercise mat with your head facing away from the wall.
2. Position yourself close to the wall, so your feet can comfortably rest against it.
3. Place your arms by your sides with your palms facing down for support.
4. Engage your core by sucking your belly button in toward your spine. This will help maintain stability throughout the exercise.
5. Inhale deeply as you press your feet against the wall to lift your hips off the mat. Your body should form a straight line from your shoulders to your knees.
6. Exhale as you reach your hips upward, engaging your glutes and core muscles. Hold this position briefly to ensure stability.
7. While maintaining the bridge position, inhale again and bring your right knee toward your chest.
8. Exhale as you use your abdominal muscles to lift your neck, shoulders, and head off the mat, reaching your forehead toward your knee. Feel the engagement in your core.
9. Inhale once more as you gently lower your head, neck, and shoulders back to the mat while extending your right leg back up toward the wall.
10. Keep your hips elevated in the bridge position.
11. Repeat the movement, but this time, bring your left knee toward your chest while inhaling deeply.
12. Exhale as you lift your head, neck, and shoulders to reach your forehead toward your left knee while keeping your hips elevated.

▶▷▶▷ ONE-LEG BRIDGE RAISE

Target: Abs and core muscles
Number of sets: 3
Repetitions per set: 20 to 30 reps (10 to 15 reps per side)

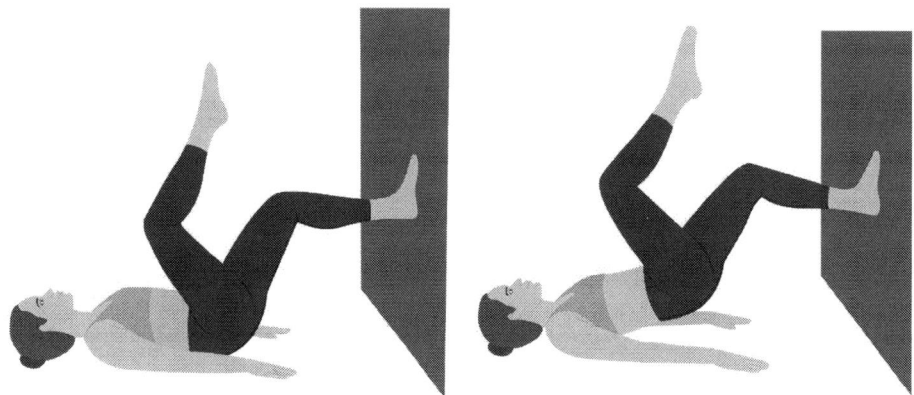

Steps

1. Begin by positioning yourself close to the wall on an exercise mat, lying on your back with your head facing away from the wall.
2. Bend your knees and place your feet flat on the wall, hip-width apart.
3. Extend your arms by your sides with your palms facing down for support.
4. Engage your core by sucking your belly button in toward your spine. This will help maintain stability throughout the movement.
5. Inhale deeply as you lift your right foot off the wall, extending your leg straight upward toward the ceiling. Your left foot remains securely planted on the wall.
6. Exhale as you press through your left heel to elevate your hips off the mat, creating a straight line from your shoulders to your left knee.
7. Focus on maintaining your balance on your left foot and the upper part of your back on the mat.
8. Hold this one-legged bridge position for a moment, feeling the activation in your left glute and hamstring.
9. Inhale once more as you slowly lower your hips back down to the mat while keeping your right leg extended.
10. Your right foot should gently touch the wall, but your hips remain elevated.
11. Exhale as you press through your left heel again to lift your hips into the bridge position.
12. Take a short break before switching to your right leg.
13. Complete three sets in total, alternating between legs.

▶▷▶▷ KNEE TO CHEST

Target: Abs and core muscles
Number of sets: 3
Repetitions per set: 20 to 30 reps (10 to 15 reps per side)

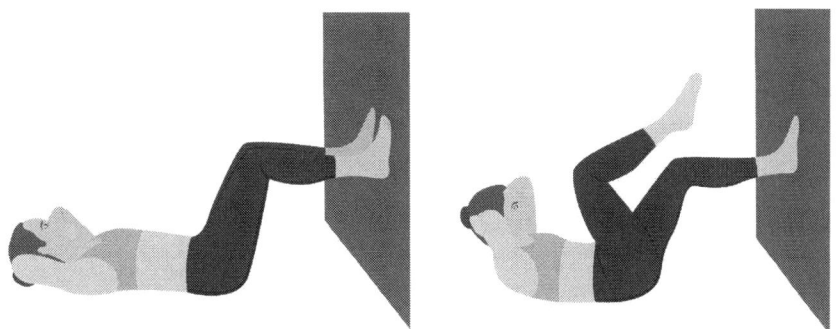

Steps

1. Begin by lying on your back on an exercise mat, facing away from the wall.
2. Position yourself close to the wall, and extend both legs vertically, gently pressing your feet against the wall.
3. Place your hands gently behind your head, taking care not to strain your neck.
4. Engage your core by sucking your belly button in toward your spine. This will help maintain stability during the movement.
5. Inhale deeply as you bend your right knee and bring it toward your chest.
6. Exhale as you use your abdominal muscles to lift your head, neck, and shoulders off the mat, reaching your forehead toward your knee.
7. Hold this position for a moment to feel the stretch and engagement in your lower abs and hip flexors.
8. Inhale again as you slowly lower your head, neck, and shoulders back to the mat.
9. Simultaneously, extend your right leg back toward the wall, resuming the initial position.
10. Repeat the movement, but this time, bend your left knee and bring it toward your chest while inhaling deeply.
11. Exhale as you lift your head, neck, and shoulders off the mat to reach your forehead toward your left knee.
12. Hold briefly to feel the stretch and contraction.
13. Alternate between your right and left legs, performing 10 to 15 repetitions for one set (5 to 7 per leg).
14. Maintain a controlled and deliberate pace throughout the exercise.
15. Take short rests between sets, and aim to complete three sets in total.

▶▷▶▷ OPPOSITE KNEE TO ELBOW

Target: Abs and core muscles
Number of sets: 3
Repetitions per set: 20 to 30 reps (10 to 15 reps per side)

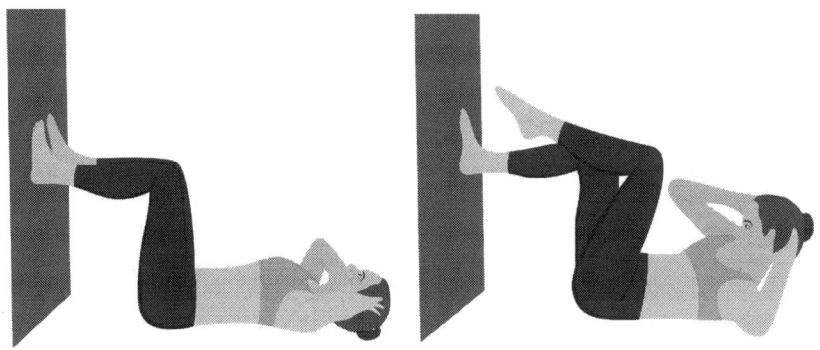

Steps

1. Begin with the basic position.
2. Bend your knees and place your feet flat on the wall, hip-width apart.
3. Place your hands on the side of your head, lightly resting them near your ears.
4. Engage your core by sucking your belly button in toward your spine. This will help maintain stability throughout the movement.
5. Inhale deeply as you lift your right foot off the wall, extending your leg straight upward toward the ceiling. Simultaneously, raise your upper body off the mat, twisting your torso to bring your left elbow toward your right knee.
6. Keep your left foot planted on the wall, while your right leg is extended and lifted.
7. Exhale as you perform this movement, aiming to touch your left elbow to your right knee.
8. Inhale again as you slowly lower your upper body and extend your right leg back to the wall. Your right foot should gently touch the wall, but your upper body remains lifted.
9. Exhale as you lift your upper body and your right leg, bringing your left elbow toward your right knee once more.
10. Continue this dynamic motion, inhaling during the lowering phase and exhaling during the lifting phase.

▶▷▶▷ 3-SECOND BEAR CRAWL

Target: Abs and core muscles
Number of sets: 3
Repetitions per set: 10 to 15 reps

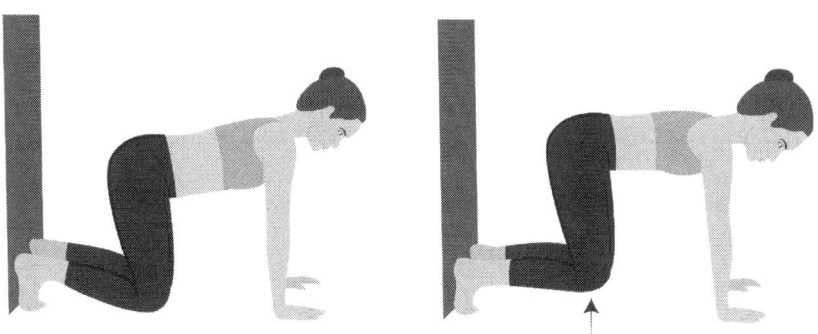

Steps

1. Begin in a downward dog position on the floor, with your hands shoulder-width apart and your palms flat on the ground.
2. Ensure your knees are touching the ground but not quite, maintaining a hover.
3. Position yourself facing away from the wall, allowing your feet to rest against the wall for support.
4. Engage your core by sucking your belly button in toward your spine. This will help stabilize your body during the movement.
5. Press your feet against the wall for support and lift your knees off the ground so your body can get into a bear crawl position.
6. Hold this position for precisely 3 seconds while keeping your core engaged and your knees hovering.
7. Exhale slowly as you release the pressure from your feet against the wall and return to the initial bear crawl position with your knees hovering above the ground.
8. Keep your core engaged throughout the movement.
9. Inhale again as you initiate the next repetition by pressing your feet against the wall, entering the bear crawl position with wall support.
10. Maintain the position for 3 seconds, focusing on stability and core engagement while ensuring your knees stay off the ground.
11. Exhale as you release the wall support and return to the initial bear crawl position with your knees hovering.

12. Continue the exercise, inhaling during the bear crawl hold and exhaling during the return to the initial position.
13. Take a brief break to catch your breath and reset.
14. Repeat the exercise for a total of three sets, maintaining proper form and controlled movements throughout.

▶▷▶▷ CAT-CAMEL

Target: Abs, back, and core muscles
Number of sets: 3
Repetitions per set: 10 to 15 reps

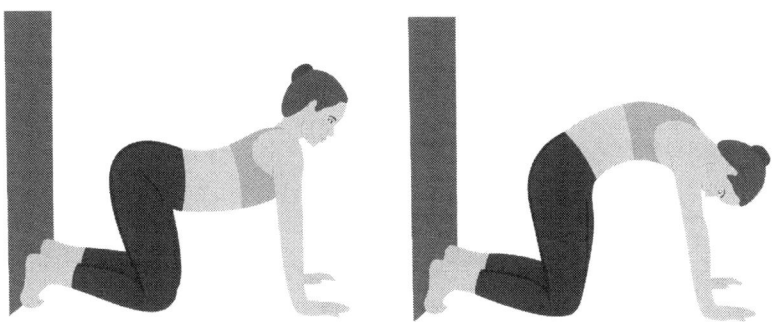

Steps

1. Begin in an all-fours position with your hands placed shoulder-width apart on the floor.
2. Position yourself facing away from the wall, ensuring that your feet are close to the wall.
3. Maintain a neutral spine with your back in a flat, tabletop position.
4. Engage your core by sucking your belly button in toward your spine. This will help stabilize your spine during the movement.
5. Inhale deeply as you initiate the Cat position: Arch your back upward toward the ceiling, tucking your chin toward your chest.
6. Simultaneously, press your feet gently against the wall to assist in lifting your pelvis slightly higher. This will create a deeper stretch in your back.
7. Hold the Cat position for a few seconds, maintaining the engagement of your core and feeling the stretch in your back.
8. Exhale slowly as you transition into the Camel position: Arch your back in the opposite direction, lowering your belly and lifting your head and tailbone upward.
9. Simultaneously, release the pressure from your feet against the wall, allowing your pelvis to lower naturally.
10. Hold the Camel position for a few seconds, focusing on the stretch in your spine and the engagement of your core muscles.
11. Inhale again as you return to the Cat position by arching your back upward and pressing your feet against the wall.
12. Hold the Cat position for a few seconds.

13. Exhale as you transition back to the Camel position, lowering your belly and releasing the pressure from your feet against the wall.
14. Hold the Camel position for a few seconds
15. Continue to flow between the Cat and Camel positions with controlled, rhythmic movements, inhaling during the Cat position and exhaling during the Camel position.

▶▷▶▷ SIDE PLANK RAISES

Target: Abs, back, and core muscles
Number of sets: 3 per side
Repetitions per set: 10 to 15 reps per side

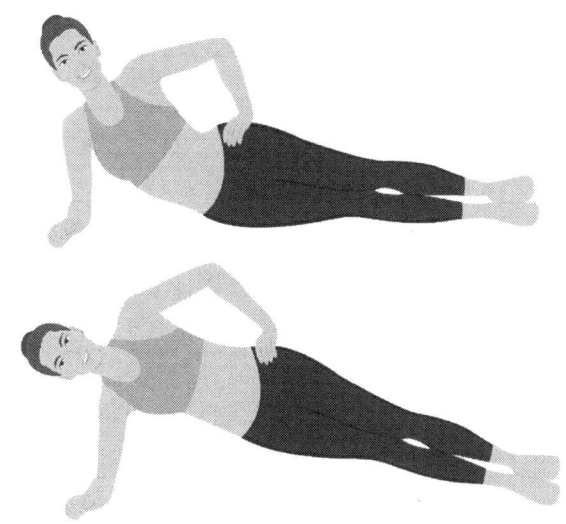

Steps

1. Begin by standing parallel to the wall, about an arm's length away from it.
2. Place your feet together and your right side facing the wall.
3. Ensure your body is in a straight line, with your head, shoulders, hips, and feet aligned.
4. Extend your right arm and place your right palm firmly against the wall at shoulder height.
5. Keep your fingers pointing forward, pressing into the wall for stability.
6. Your left hand can rest on your left hip or be extended toward the ceiling.
7. Inhale deeply as you engage your core muscles.
8. On the exhale, lift your hips off the ground while maintaining a straight line from head to heels.
9. Focus on using your core strength to support your body in the side plank position.
10. Keep your left arm extended or resting on your left hip throughout this phase.
11. Inhale again and begin the movement: Slowly lower your hips back down toward the ground.
12. Just before your hips touch the floor, exhale and raise them back up to the side plank position.
13. Ensure your movements are controlled and deliberate.
14. Perform 10 to 15 repetitions on your right side before switching to the left side.
15. To switch sides, turn around so your left side faces the wall.
16. Place your left palm on the wall for support and raise your hips into a side plank.
17. After working both sides, take a short break to reset.

▶▷▶▷ INCLINED SINGLE LEG CRUNCH (INCLINE BICYCLE CRUNCH)

Target: Abs and core muscles
Number of sets: 3
Repetitions per set: 20 to 30 reps (10 to 15 reps per leg)

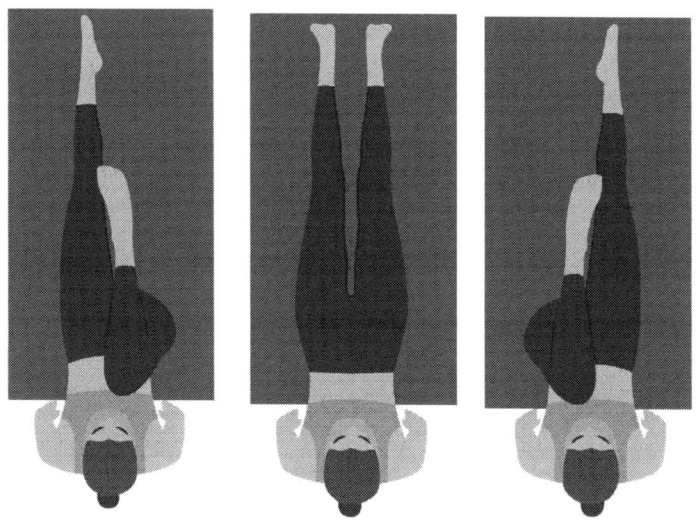

Steps

1. Begin by positioning yourself on the floor, facing the wall with your back to it.
2. Lie down with your lower back pressed against the wall.
3. Extend your legs fully, resting them against the wall.
4. Place your arms flat on the ground, palms touching the ground for support.
5. Step 2: Lift Your Upper Body
6. On the exhale, lift your upper body off the floor, aiming to bring your right elbow toward your left knee.
7. As you crunch up, simultaneously lift your left leg off the wall and bring your right elbow closer to your left knee.
8. In a twisting motion, bring your left elbow closer to your right knee while extending your right leg outward. Imagine you're pedaling a bicycle.
9. Keep your movements controlled and avoid any jerking motions.
10. Inhale again as you return to the center position with your upper body and legs.
11. Your lower back should remain in contact with the wall throughout the movement.
12. Exhale and repeat the movement, this time bringing your left elbow toward your right knee while extending your left leg.
13. Continue alternating sides with each repetition.

▶▷▶▷ V-SIT UPS

Target: Abs, hamstrings, and core muscles
Number of sets: 3
Repetitions per set: 10 to 15 reps

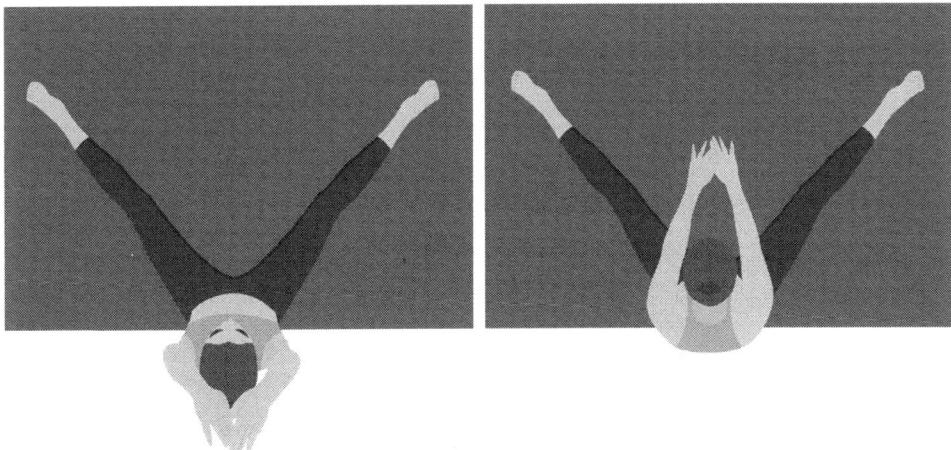

Steps

1. Begin by sitting on the floor with your back flat against it.
2. Position yourself close to a wall, ensuring that your buttocks and legs are against the wall.
3. Open your legs into a "V" shape, similar to a semi-split.
4. Place your hands on the floor beside your hips with your fingers pointing toward your toes.
5. Take a deep breath in and engage your core muscles, pressing your lower back firmly against the floor.
6. As you exhale, lift your upper body off the ground, aiming to touch your chest to your knees.
7. Keep your legs extended, creating a "V" shape with your thighs.
8. At the highest point of the movement, extend your arms toward your feet, reaching as far as you can.
9. This action helps intensify the engagement of your abdominal muscles.
10. Maintain the V-Sit Up position for a brief moment, concentrating on contracting your core muscles.
11. Ensure stability and balance during this phase.
12. Inhale as you gently lower your upper body back down to the initial position.
13. Control the descent and avoid letting your back arch off the floor.
14. Exhale and repeat the V-Sit Up movement, raising your upper body and aiming for the V position with your legs against the wall.
15. Execute the exercise with steady and controlled motions.

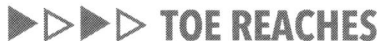 **TOE REACHES**

Target: Abs, hamstrings, and core muscles
Number of sets: 3
Repetitions per set: 10 to 15 reps

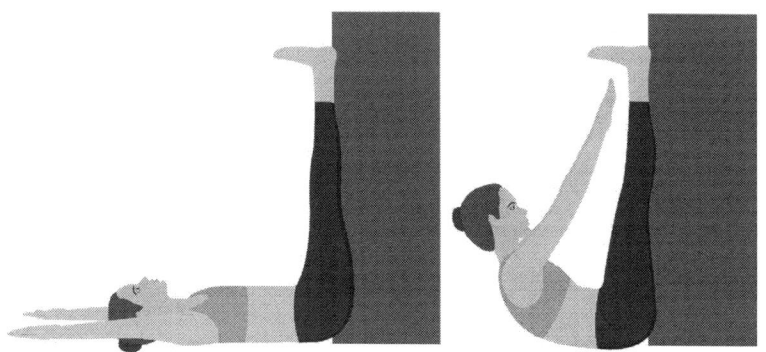

Steps

1. Begin by lying on your back on the floor with your legs extended upward, resting against the wall.
2. Your legs should be vertical against the wall, forming a 90-degree angle with the floor.
3. Extend your arms forward, reaching them straight up toward your toes.
4. Your arms should remain parallel to each other throughout the exercise.
5. Take a deep breath in, engaging your core muscles by drawing your navel toward your spine.
6. This engagement will provide stability and support for your lower back.
7. As you exhale, slowly lift your upper body off the floor, aiming to reach your toes with your fingertips.
8. Keep your arms straight and parallel during this movement.
9. Focus on using your abdominal muscles to lift your upper body.
10. Continue reaching upward with your arms while trying to touch your toes with your fingertips.
11. Maintain a controlled and deliberate motion throughout this phase.
12. Hold the position for a brief moment at the peak of the movement, ensuring a strong contraction in your abdominal muscles.
13. Feel the stretch in your hamstrings as you reach toward your toes.
14. Inhale as you slowly lower your upper body back down to the initial position, one vertebra at a time.
15. Keep your core engaged to prevent any jerky or uncontrolled movements.
16. Exhale and repeat the Toe Reach movement, lifting your upper body and reaching toward your toes.

CHAPTER 4: IMPROVING BACK POSTURE

Have you ever experienced those nagging aches and pains in your lower back, shoulders, or neck? It's often a result of not paying enough attention to your posture.

Whether you spend long hours standing or sitting, work on a laptop that's not at eye level, or constantly find yourself looking down at your phone, these habits can seriously impact your posture and well-being. But fear not, as the right exercises can make a world of difference.

In a recent survey done online by Vasileios Korakakis et al. (February 2019) involving 544 skilled female physiotherapists, a staggering 93.9% of the participants stressed the significance of educating women about maintaining optimal sitting and standing postures.

The findings revealed that 97.5% and 98.2% of these professionals highlighted three distinct sitting positions and two different standing postures as ideal.

These preferred postures consistently emphasized an upright and well-aligned stance, aligning perfectly with our journey towards better posture through Wall Pilates.

Workouts

▶▷▶▷ WALL PUSH-UPS

Target: Upper body, back, chest, and arms
Number of sets: 3
Repetitions per set: 10 to 15 reps

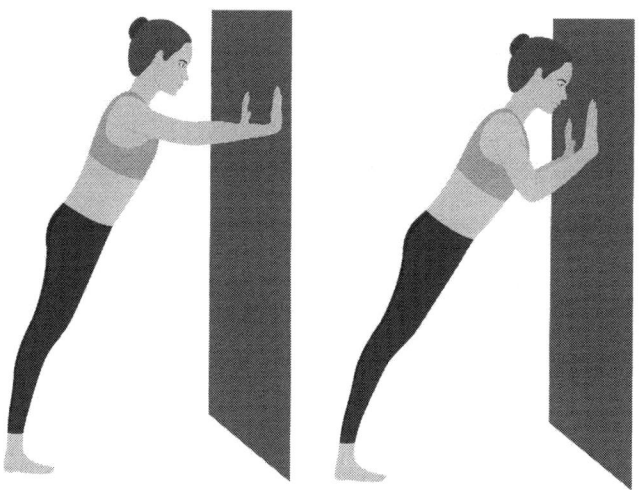

Steps

1. Stand facing a sturdy wall, approximately arm's length away.
2. Place your feet hip-width apart and keep them firmly planted on the ground.
3. Extend your arms in front of you and raise them to shoulder level.
4. Place your palms flat on the wall, with your hands slightly wider than shoulder-width apart.
5. Your fingers should be pointing straight ahead or slightly turned outward.
6. Ensure that your body forms a straight line from your head to your heels. Maintain a neutral spine throughout the exercise.
7. Engage your core muscles by drawing your navel toward your spine to provide stability.
8. Inhale as you bend your elbows and slowly lean your upper body toward the wall.
9. Keep your elbows close to your body as you lower yourself.
10. Continue lowering your chest toward the wall until your nose is just a few inches away from it.
11. Maintain a controlled and deliberate motion throughout the descent.
12. Your feet should remain flat on the ground.
13. Exhale as you push your body away from the wall by straightening your arms.
14. Focus on using your chest and arm muscles to lift your body back to the starting position.

▶▷▶▷ ONE ARM WALL PUSH-UPS

Target: Upper body, back, chest, and arms
Number of sets: 3
Repetitions per set: 10 to 15 reps (per arm)

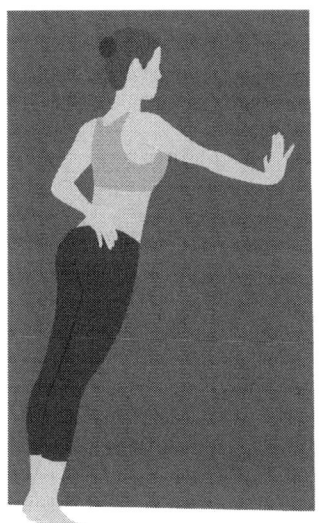 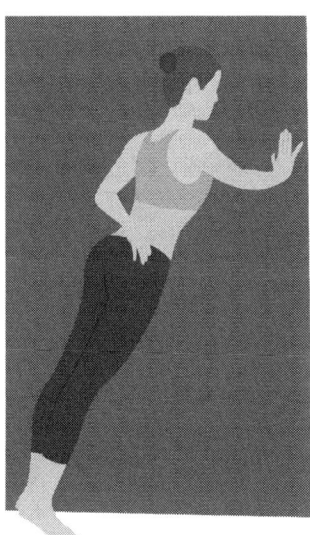

Steps

1. Stand facing the wall, approximately an arm's length away, with your feet hip-width apart.
2. Extend both of your arms straight out in front of you, placing your palms flat against the wall at shoulder height, with your fingers pointing upward. This serves as your starting position.
3. Take a slight step back from the wall, creating a slight angle between your upper body and the wall. Ensure that your head, shoulders, hips, and heels form a straight line.
4. Engage your core muscles to maintain a stable and straight body alignment.
5. Initiate the exercise by lifting your left hand off the wall while keeping your right hand firmly in place. Your right arm should now be extended straight out in front of you.
6. Place your left hand on the small of your back, just above your buttocks, elbow bent at 90 degrees.
7. Hold this position for a moment, focusing on engaging your core to prevent any twisting or tilting of your body.
8. Do a push up by lowering your upper body towards the wall, and push yourself back to the upright position.
9. Do 10 to 15 reps before swapping your right arm before switching to your left.
10. Be mindful and execute this exercise with control, emphasizing balance and stability, all while maintaining the one-arm push-up position against the wall.

▶▷▶▷ PLANK SHOULDER TAPS

Target: Core muscles, including the rectus abdominis and obliques, as well as your shoulder muscles
Number of sets: 3
Repetitions per set: 20 to 30 reps (10 - 15 taps per side)

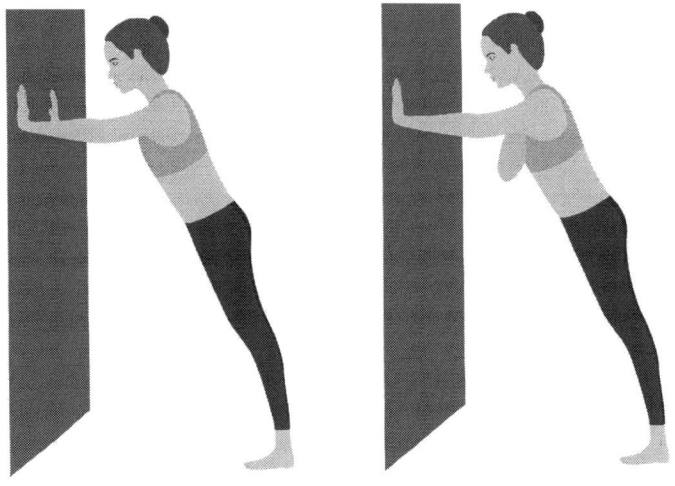

Steps

1. Begin by facing the wall and placing your hands firmly against it, at shoulder height. Your arms should be fully extended, and your fingers should point upward.
2. Step your feet back so that your body forms a straight line from your head to your heels. Engage your core muscles to maintain this straight alignment.
3. Lift your right hand off the wall and reach it across your body to touch your left shoulder. Focus on keeping your hips as stable as possible during this movement.
4. Carefully return your right hand to the wall, then raise your left hand off the wall and reach it across to touch your right shoulder.
5. Alternate between touching your shoulders with your hands while concentrating on keeping your core engaged to prevent any swaying or twisting of your hips.
6. Execute this exercise in a controlled manner, emphasizing balance and stability. Avoid rushing through the movements.

▶▷▶▷ ELBOW TO PLANK

Target: Core muscles, including the rectus abdominis and obliques, as well as your shoulder muscles
Number of sets: 3
Repetitions per set: 15 to 20 reps

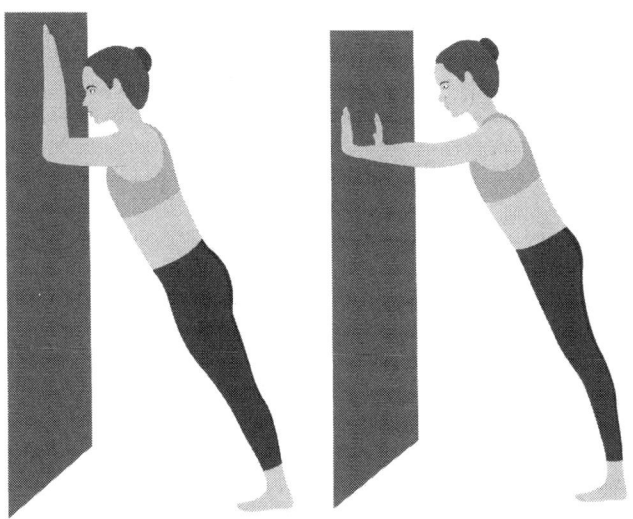

Steps

1. Stand facing the wall with your feet hip-width apart, ensuring your toes are about a foot away from the wall.
2. Place your palms and inner forearms flat against the wall, bending your elbows to 90 degrees. Your bent elbows should now align with your shoulders.
3. Step your feet back slightly, creating a slight angle between your upper body and the wall. This will be your starting position.
4. Engage your core muscles to maintain a stable and straight body alignment, ensuring your head, shoulders, hips, and heels form a straight line.
5. Begin the exercise by extending your arms straight in front of you, while keeping your palms in place on the wall. This will lift your elbows off the wall.
6. Hold this position for 20 seconds, making sure that your core remains engaged to prevent any twisting or tilting of your body.
7. Slowly return your arms to their original position on the wall to complete one repetition.
8. Aim for 15 to 20 repetitions to complete one set.

▶▷▶▷ WALL ANGELS

Target: Shoulder and back muscles
Number of sets: 3
Repetitions per set: 15 to 20 reps

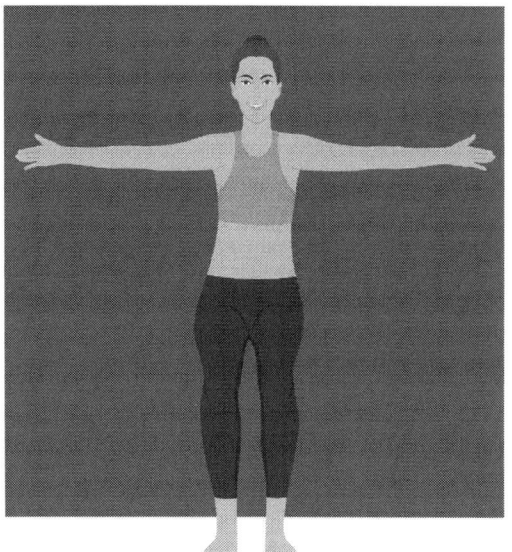 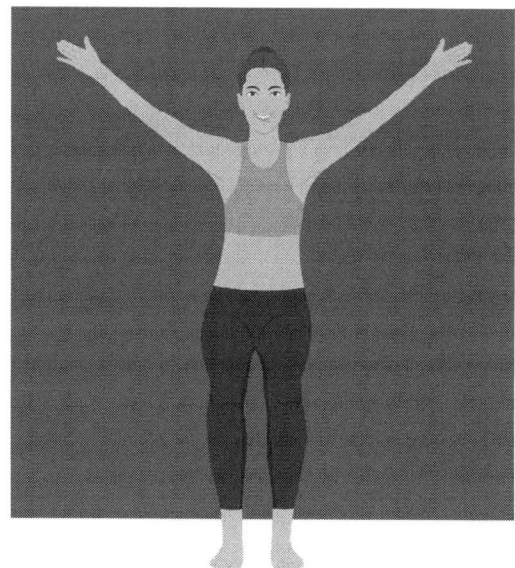

Steps

1. Stand with your back against a wall. Your feet should be about hip-width apart, and your heels, buttocks, shoulders, and head should all touch the wall. Maintain a natural arch in your lower back.
2. Extend your arms straight out to the sides, forming a "T" shape with your body. Your palms should be facing forward, and your fingertips should lightly touch the wall.
3. Inhale deeply and engage your core muscles to maintain stability.
4. Begin the movement by sliding your arms upward along the wall, keeping your palms facing forward. Imagine you are trying to touch the wall above your head.
5. As you raise your arms, make sure to keep your wrists, elbows, and shoulders in contact with the wall. Your goal is to maintain three points of contact with the wall at all times.
6. Continue to slide your arms upward as far as comfortably possible while maintaining proper form.
7. Once your arms are extended overhead, pause briefly to feel the stretch in your chest and shoulders.
8. Exhale slowly as you reverse the movement, sliding your arms back down to the starting position.
9. Throughout the exercise, focus on keeping your entire back, head, and arms in contact with the wall. This ensures that you are moving through the full range of motion.

▶▷▶▷ CHEST OPENER

Target: Back muscles and chest
Number of sets: 3
Repetitions per set: 15 to 20 reps

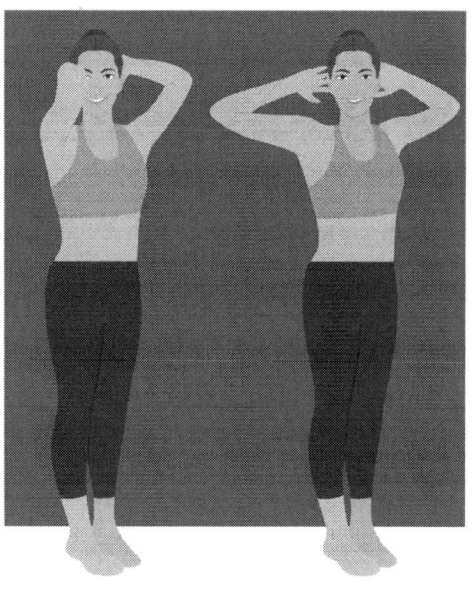

Steps

1. Stand with your back against a wall, ensuring your feet are hip-width apart. Your heels, buttocks, shoulders, and head should all touch the wall. Maintain a neutral spine with a slight natural arch in your lower back.
2. Hold your hands behind your head, inhale deeply, and engage your core muscles to maintain stability.
3. Slowly bring your forearms forward, allowing them to meet at the center of your chest while keeping them perpendicular to the floor. Your fingertips should lightly touch the wall as you cross your forearms.
4. As you cross your forearms, feel a gentle stretch in your chest and shoulders. Hold this stretched position for a moment while continuing to breathe deeply.
5. Exhale slowly as you return your forearms back to the starting position with control, keeping them perpendicular to the floor.
6. Throughout the exercise, focus on keeping your entire back, head, and forearms in contact with the wall. This ensures that you are moving through the full range of motion.

▶▷▶▷ SHOULDER PRESS

Target: Back muscles
Number of sets: 3
Repetitions per set: 15 to 20 reps

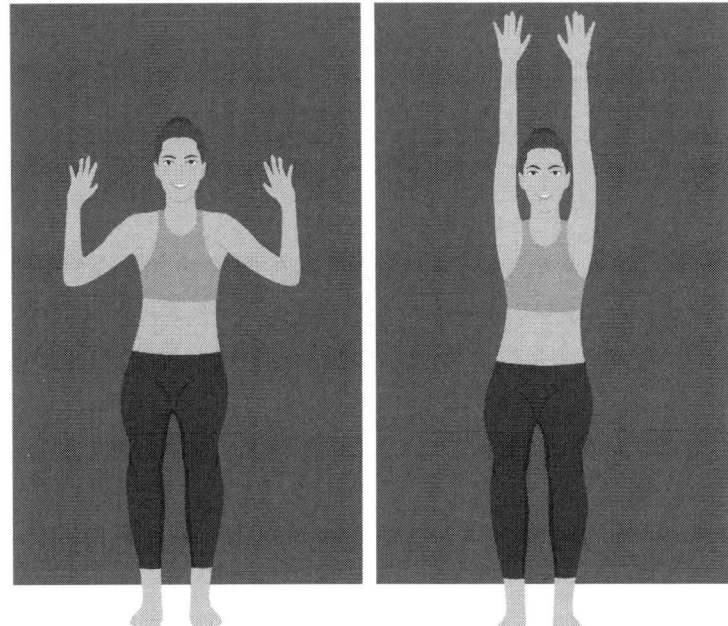

Steps

1. Stand with your back against a wall, ensuring your feet are hip-width apart. Your heels, buttocks, shoulders, and head should all touch the wall. Maintain a neutral spine with a slight natural arch in your lower back.
2. Start with your arms bent at 45 degrees and your forearms are parallel to the floor. Your palms should be facing forward, and your fingertips should lightly touch the wall.
3. Inhale deeply and engage your core muscles to maintain stability.
4. Exhale as you press your arms up and away from the wall, straightening them fully while keeping your forearms parallel to the floor. This movement mimics the action of pressing something heavy overhead.
5. At the top of the movement, your arms should be fully extended, and your hands should lightly touch the wall above your head.
6. Inhale as you slowly lower your arms back to the starting position with control, maintaining the 90-degree bend in your elbows.
7. Throughout the exercise, focus on keeping your entire back, head, and arms in contact with the wall. This ensures that you are moving through the full range of motion.

▶▷▶▷ ISOMETRIC PULLS

Target: Back muscles and chest
Number of sets: 3
Repetitions per set: 15 to 20 reps

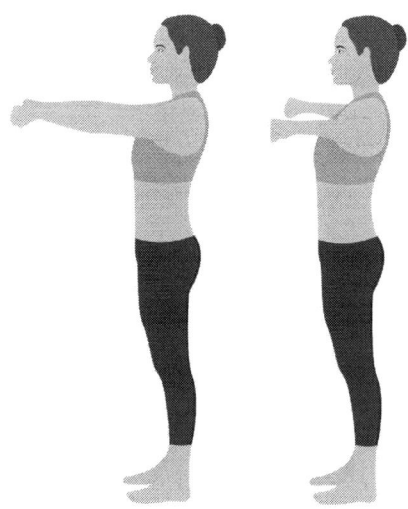

Steps

1. Start by standing with your back against the wall, ensuring your feet are hip-width apart and your toes are pointing forward.
2. Position yourself so that your nose, chest, and knees are all in line with each other. Maintain a neutral spine with a slight natural arch in your lower back.
3. Extend your arms straight in front of you at shoulder height, parallel to the floor and your fists should slightly touch the wall.
4. Inhale deeply, engaging your core muscles to stabilize your body.
5. Exhale as you initiate the isometric pull. Imagine pulling your shoulder blades together against the wall using your upper back muscles. While doing this, maintain the position of your arms and keep them at shoulder height.
6. Focus on squeezing your shoulder blades together as you hold the pull against the wall for a few seconds. Feel the engagement in your upper back.
7. Inhale as you release the isometric pull, and return to the starting position with your arms extended straight ahead.

▶▷▶▷ DIAMOND PUSH-UPS

Target: Back muscles, triceps, and chest
Number of sets: 3
Repetitions per set: 15 to 20 reps

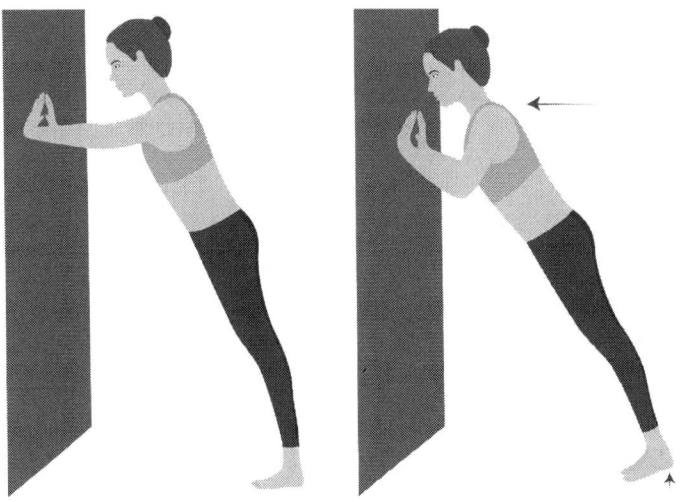

Steps

1. Stand facing the wall, approximately arm's length away.
2. Place your hands on the wall, close together, forming a diamond shape with your thumbs and index fingers. Your fingers should be pointing upward.
3. Step your feet back slightly, creating a diagonal line from your head to your heels. Keep your core engaged and your body in a straight line.
4. Inhale deeply as you lower your chest toward the wall. Keep your elbows close to your body as you descend.
5. Exhale and push against the wall to return to the starting position, fully extending your arms. Keep your body in a straight line throughout the movement.
6. Continue to perform diamond pushups, inhaling as you lower your chest and exhaling as you push back up.

▶▷▶▷ **DECLINE PUSH UPS**

Target: Chest, shoulders, triceps, and core.
Number of sets: 3
Repetitions per set: 7 to 10 reps

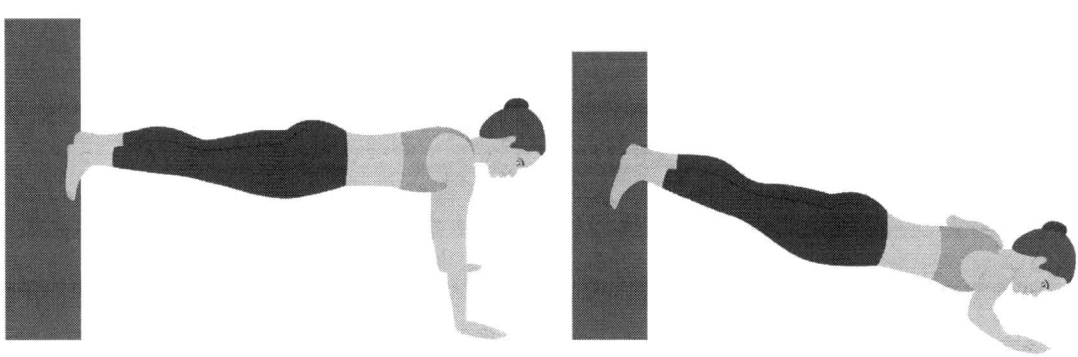

Steps

1. Position Yourself: Start by facing away from the wall, about an arm's length away. Place your hands on the floor slightly wider than shoulder-width apart, fingers pointing forward.
2. Wall Placement: Extend your legs and place the soles of your feet against the wall, creating an inclined angle with your body. The higher your feet on the wall, the more challenging the exercise will be.
3. Engage Your Core: Inhale deeply and engage your core muscles. Your body should form a straight line from head to heels.
4. Begin the Push-Up: Exhale as you lower your chest toward the floor by bending your elbows. Keep your body in a straight line throughout the movement.
5. Lower to Your Comfort Level: Lower yourself until your chest is about an inch or two from the floor or to your comfort level. Ensure your elbows are at a 90-degree angle or slightly less.
6. Push Back Up: Push through your palms and exhale as you extend your arms, returning to the starting position. Keep your body straight throughout the motion.
7. Repeat the Push-Ups: Continue performing push-ups for the desired number of repetitions, maintaining good form and core engagement.
8. Rest Between Sets: After completing one set, take a brief rest before starting the next set. Aim to complete three sets.

▶▷▶▷ SHOULDER FRONT RAISES

Target: Front deltoids (front shoulder muscles).
Number of sets: 3
Repetitions per set: 10 to 15 reps

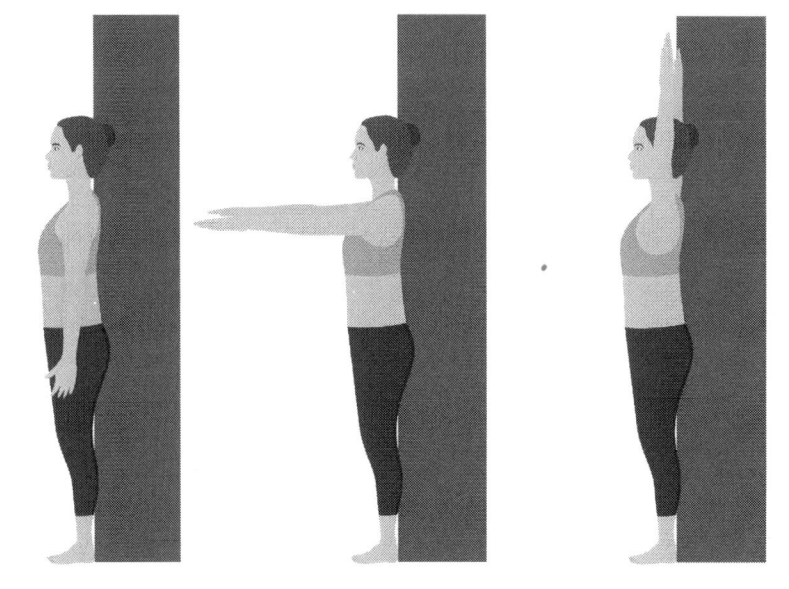

Steps

1. Stand with your back against the wall. Stand up straight with your feet hip-width apart. Your toes should be pointing forward.
2. Extend your arms straight in front of you, parallel to the floor.
3. Inhale deeply and engage your core muscles to stabilize your body.
4. Exhale as you slowly lift your arms upward while keeping them straight. Your goal is to raise your arms above your head. Make sure you are comfortable and that your shoulders have no strain or discomfort.
5. As you lift your arms, focus on controlled and deliberate movements. Avoid any swinging or jerking motions.
6. When your arms reach the desired height, pause for a moment to engage your front shoulder muscles.
7. Inhale as you slowly lower your arms back to the starting position against the wall, maintaining control throughout the descent.
8. Continue performing front raises for the desired number of repetitions, maintaining good form and core engagement.
9. After completing one set, take a brief rest before starting the next set. Aim to complete three sets.

▶▷▶▷ LEG CURLS

Target: Back, core, and hamstrings
Number of sets: 3
Repetitions per set: 10 to 15 reps

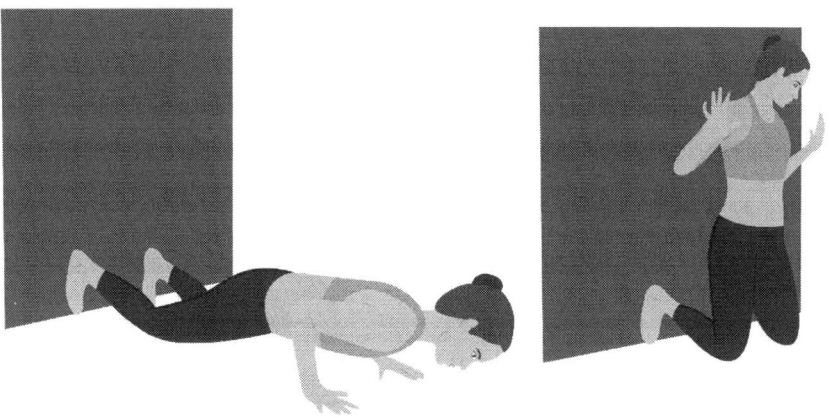

Steps

1. Begin by kneeling down on your hands and knees, facing away from the wall. Your hands should be on the floor, and your knees should be directly under your hips.
2. Extend both of your legs straight behind you, pressing the soles of your feet against the wall. Your toes should be in contact with the ground to maintain stability.
3. While keeping your feet on the wall, walk your hands slightly wider than shoulder-width apart, positioning them at the same level as your shoulders.
4. Bend your elbows to lower your upper body into a push-up position. Your shoulders should be in line with your hips, creating a straight line from head to heels.
5. Exhale as you use the strength of your upper body, hamstrings, and core muscles to push the ground away. Simultaneously, pull your feet toward your glutes by bending your knees.
6. As your knees curl in and your feet move closer to your glutes, lift your upper body away from the floor. Your goal is to create a smooth, flowing motion as you curl your legs and lift your upper body.
7. Keep your shoulders in line with your hips throughout the movement, maintaining proper form.
8. Inhale as you use your hamstrings and core muscles to slowly and control lower your upper body back to the starting position, resembling a push-up position.

▶▷▶▷ TOE TOUCHES

Target: Abdominals (especially the lower abs), hip flexors, and quadriceps
Number of sets: 3
Repetitions per set: 10 to 15 reps

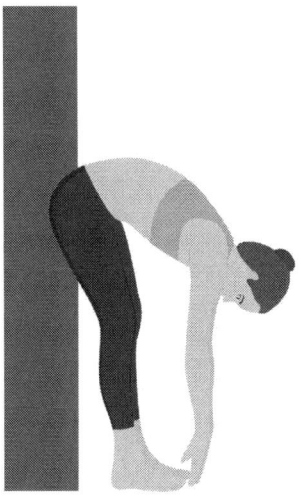

Steps

1. Stand with your back against the wall, ensuring your feet are hip-width apart.
2. Gently press your lower back against the wall. This maintains contact with the wall while engaging your core.
3. Extend your arms straight up toward the ceiling, keeping them close to your ears. Your palms should be facing forward.
4. Inhale deeply and engage your core muscles.
5. As you exhale, bring your upper body and extend your arms forward and downward. You're aiming to touch your hands to your toes.
6. Reach as far as your flexibility allows, but don't force the movement. If you can't touch your toes, that's perfectly fine.
7. Return your upper body and arms to the upright position against the wall to complete the repetition.
8. Continue the repetitions for the desired number of repetitions. Each toe touch counts as one rep.
9. After completing one set, take a brief rest before starting the next set. Aim to complete three sets.

CHAPTER 5. SHAPING THE BUTTOCKS

In the world of Pilates, the glutes—the often-neglected but mighty muscles of the buttocks—are a crucial component of the "powerhouse." This powerhouse encompasses the muscles in your abs, lower back, pelvic floor, hips, and yes, your lovely behind. What's fascinating about Pilates is that it's all about deliberate, controlled movements, which means you engage not only the major muscles but also the smaller, supportive ones that tend to get overlooked.

The beauty of Wall Pilates lies in its simplicity; you don't need fancy gym equipment or heavy weights to target and tone those glutes. Pilates offers a safe and effective way to work on your booty, favored by celebrities like Cameron Diaz, Kate Hudson, and Jennifer Aniston. What sets Pilates apart is its emphasis on proper form and controlled movements, reducing the risk of injury that can be associated with traditional gym exercises.

Traditional exercises like squats, lunges, and leg presses can sometimes lead to injuries, especially if your glutes are not firing correctly, and your quads take over. Wall Pilates for the buttocks offers a safer alternative, ensuring your glutes are the stars of the show, without risking harm to your spine or other muscle groups.

In this chapter, we will explore a series of Wall Pilates exercises designed to target and strengthen your glutes, helping you achieve the sculpted and toned booty you desire. Get ready to embark on a journey of controlled movements and controlled results, all while prioritizing the safety and effectiveness of your workout. Let's dive in and give your glutes the attention they deserve!

Workouts

▶▷▶▷ KICK BACKS

Target: Glutes and back
Number of sets: 3
Repetitions per set: 20 to 30 reps (10 - 15 reps per leg)

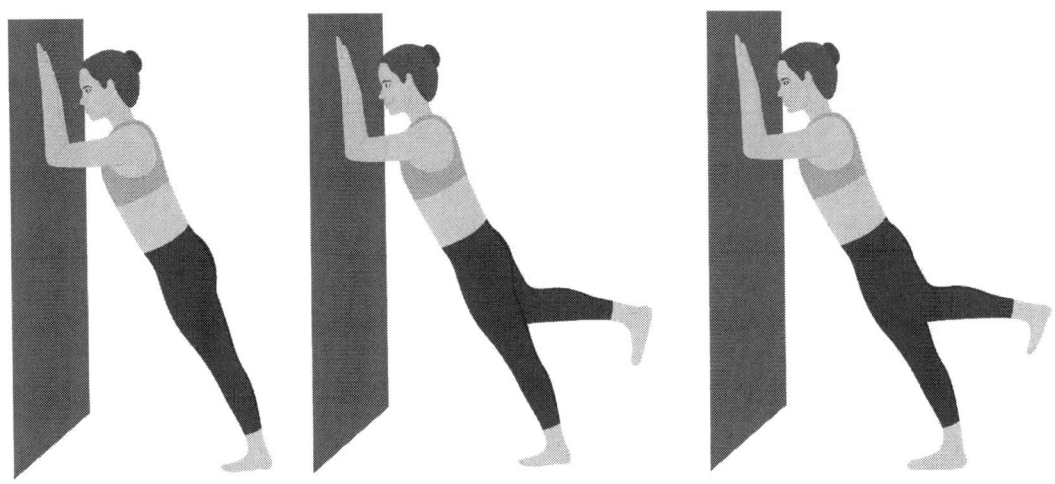

Steps

1. Begin by standing with your feet hip-width apart, facing the wall. Your toes should be pointing forward.
2. Place your palms on the wall at shoulder height, with your arms extended straight. For a more challenging workout, bend your elbows, and rest your forearms flat against the wall.
3. Engage your core muscles to stabilize your spine.
4. Shift your weight to your left leg while keeping your right foot on the ground for balance.
5. Slowly lift your right leg behind you, keeping it straight, and engage your glutes throughout the movement. Your foot should be flexed, and your toes should be pointing toward the floor.
6. Lift your right leg as high as comfortable, without arching your lower back. You should feel your glutes contracting.
7. Hold the raised position for a brief moment, focusing on squeezing your glutes.
8. Lower your right leg back to the starting position, but don't let it touch the ground between repetitions.

▶▷▶▷ SPLIT SQUATS

Target: Glutes, quadriceps, hamstrings, calves
Number of sets: 3
Repetitions per set: 20 to 30 reps (10 - 15 reps per leg)

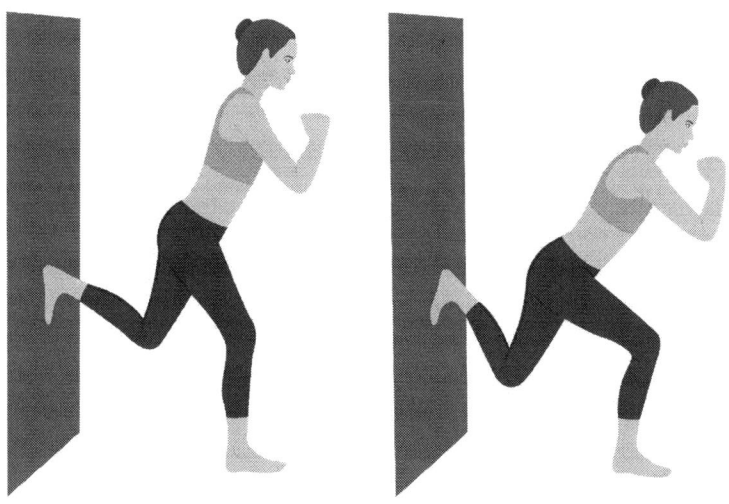

Steps

1. Stand with your back against a wall, and your feet hip-width apart. Your heels should be about a foot's length away from the wall. If you're using a yoga mat, place it on the floor for added comfort.
2. Extend your right leg straight behind you and place the top of your right foot flat against the wall. Your toes should point down towards the ground.
3. Make sure your left knee is directly above your left ankle, forming a 90-degree angle with your left thigh parallel to the floor. This is your starting position.
4. Slowly lower your body into a lunge by bending your left knee. Keep your upper body upright and your back against the wall. As you descend, your right knee should come close to, but not touch, the ground.
5. Push through your left heel to return to the starting position. Focus on engaging your glutes and quads as you rise.
6. Complete the desired number of reps for your left leg, then switch to your right leg. Extend your left leg back and place the top of your left foot against the wall, toes pointing down.
7. Throughout the exercise, keep your core engaged, shoulders relaxed, and gaze straight ahead. Remember to breathe evenly throughout the movement.

▶▷▶▷ WALL SQUATS

Target: Glutes, quadriceps, hamstrings, and calves.
Number of sets: 3
Repetitions per set: 10 - 15 reps

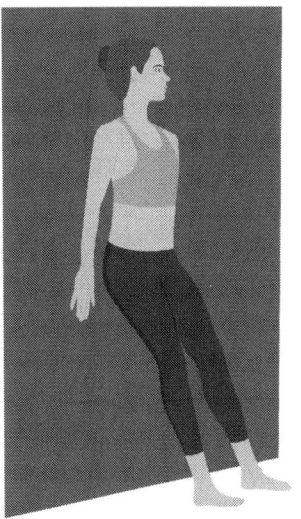 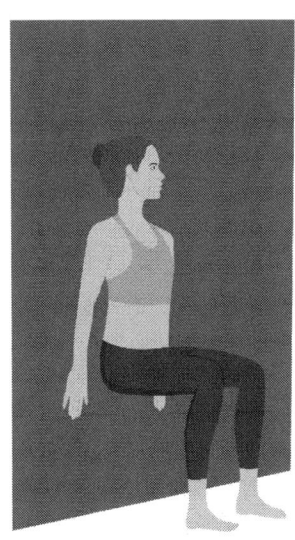

Steps

1. Begin by standing with your back against a wall. Ensure your feet are hip-width apart and about 12 to 18 inches away from the wall. Your feet should be parallel to each other.
2. Tighten your abdominal muscles to engage your core. This will help support your lower back throughout the exercise.
3. Slowly begin to lower your body by bending your knees. Imagine you're sitting back in an invisible chair. Keep your back against the wall as you descend.
4. Lower your body with control until your knees are bent at approximately a 90-degree angle. Your thighs should be parallel to the floor or as close as comfortable. Your knees should align with your ankles, not extending beyond them.
5. Ensure that your back remains in contact with the wall throughout the movement. Focus on keeping your chest up and your shoulders relaxed.
6. Be mindful of your knee position; they should be pointing straight ahead, tracking in line with your toes. Avoid letting your knees collapse inward.
7. Once you've reached the lowest point of your squat, hold this position for a moment. Take a deep breath in and exhale slowly.
8. Push through your heels and engage your glutes and quadriceps to rise back up to the starting position. Keep your back against the wall as you ascend.

▶▷▶▷ WALL SIT (WALL SQUAT HOLD)

Target: Glutes, quadriceps, hamstrings, and calves.
Number of sets: 3
Repetitions per set: 30 - 60 seconds each set

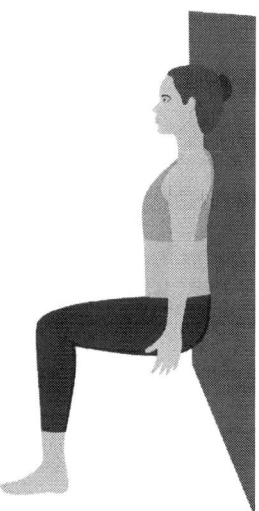

Steps

1. Stand with your back against a wall. Your feet should be about hip-width apart and positioned slightly in front of you.
2. Ensure your feet are parallel to each other and your heels are about 12 to 18 inches away from the wall.
3. Slowly lower your body into a squat position by bending your knees. Imagine you're sitting back in an invisible chair.
4. Keep your back firmly against the wall throughout the exercise. This is essential for proper form and support.
5. Your knees should be in line with your ankles, not extending past them. Aim to get your thighs parallel to the floor, if possible.
6. Engage your core muscles to maintain stability, and keep your chest lifted.
7. As you hold the squat position, focus on your breath. Take slow, deep breaths to stay relaxed and maintain good form.
8. Continue to hold the squat for the desired duration, starting with 30 seconds and gradually working your way up to 60 seconds or more as you become more comfortable.
9. To exit the squat, slowly push through your heels, straightening your legs and returning to a standing position.
10. Take a moment to stretch your legs and shake them out if needed.

▶▷▶▷ FORWARD WALL SQUAT

Target: Glutes, quadriceps, hamstrings, and calves.
Number of sets: 3
Repetitions per set: 10 - 15 reps

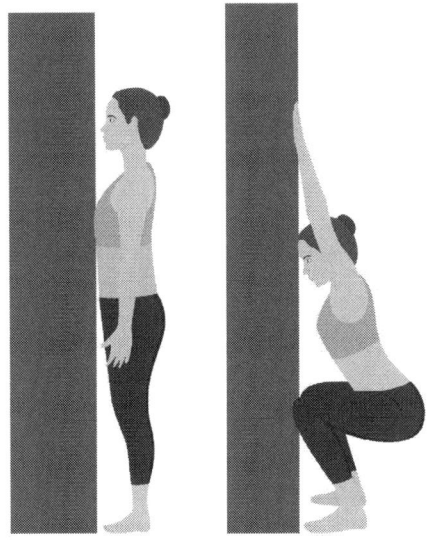

Steps

1. Stand facing the wall with your feet together and your toes touching the wall–if you are able to. Your heels should be about hip-width apart.
2. Place your hands on the wall at shoulder height or slightly higher for support.
3. Keep your chest lifted and your back straight. Engage your core muscles to maintain stability.
4. Slowly lower your body into a squat position by bending your knees. Imagine you're sitting back in an invisible chair.
5. As you lower yourself, your knees will naturally move forward, touching the wall. Keep your knees in line with your ankles.
6. Your goal is to lower yourself until your thighs are parallel to the floor, or as close to parallel as your flexibility allows.
7. Ensure your weight is evenly distributed across both feet, with your heels on the ground.
8. Hold the squat position for a moment to engage your glutes and thighs.
9. Push through your heels to stand back up, straightening your legs and returning to the starting position.

▶▷▶▷ ONE-LEGGED WALL SQUATS

Target: Glutes, quadriceps, hamstrings, calves
Number of sets: 3
Repetitions per set: 10 to 12 reps (5 - 6 reps per leg)

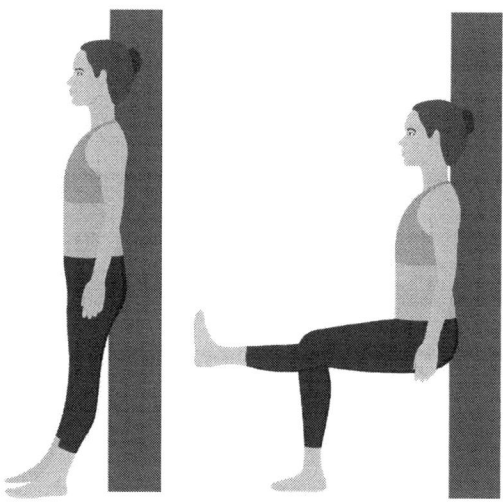

Steps

1. Stand with your back against the wall.
2. Lower your upper body down into the squat position so your thighs are no more than 90 degrees with the floor.
3. Place your hands on the wall, parallel to you shoulder, on either side of your hips for support.
4. Keep your chest lifted and your back straight. Engage your core muscles to maintain stability.
5. Now shift your weight to your left leg, raising your right leg straight out in front of you.
6. Hold the squat position for a moment to engage your glutes and thighs.
7. Push through your left heel to stand back up, placing your right leg back on the floor and returning to the upright position.
8. Repeat the above steps, shifting your weight to your right leg and lifting your left leg off the floor.
9. Repeat this movement for the desired number of repetitions, starting with 10 to 15 reps per leg.

▶▷▶▷ LATERAL LEG SWINGS

Target: Glutes, quadriceps, hamstrings, calves
Number of sets: 3
Repetitions per set: 20 to 30 reps (10 - 15 reps per leg)

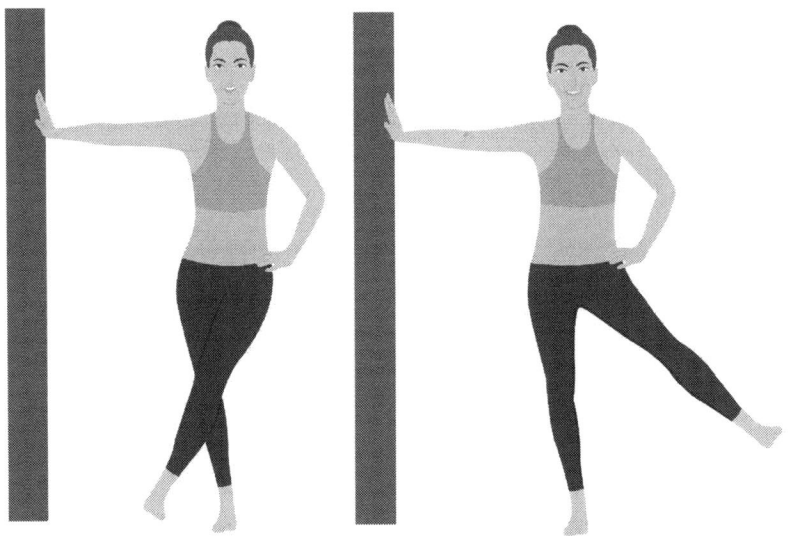

Steps

1. Stand sideways to the wall with your right side facing the wall. Place one hand on the wall for balance and support.
2. Keep your feet together and your toes pointing forward.
3. Engage your core muscles to maintain stability and good posture throughout the exercise.
4. Shift your weight onto your right leg while keeping your left foot relaxed and off the ground.
5. Begin to swing your left leg to the side away from the wall in a controlled manner. Keep your leg straight but not locked at the knee.
6. Swing your left leg as high as comfortably possible to the side without leaning your upper body or losing balance.
7. Slowly swing your left leg back toward the wall to its starting position without letting it touch the ground.
8. Repeat this swinging motion for the desired number of repetitions, starting with 10 to 15 swings for your left leg.
9. Switch to your right side to perform the same number of swings for balance and symmetry.

▶▷▶▷ FORWARD LEG SWINGS

Target: Glutes, hip flexors, and quadriceps
Number of sets: 3
Repetitions per set: 20 to 30 reps (10 - 15 reps per leg)

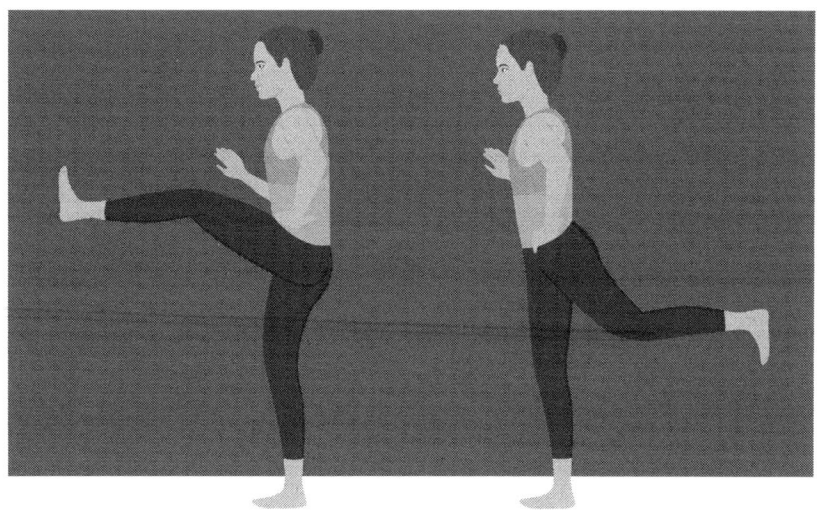

Steps

1. Stand parallel to the wall, so that your side/shoulder is facing the wall with your feet hip-width apart. Place one hand on the wall for balance and support.
2. Keep your posture tall, shoulders relaxed, and core engaged throughout the exercise.
3. Begin by shifting your weight onto your right leg while keeping your left foot relaxed and off the ground.
4. Swing your left leg forward in a controlled manner, aiming to raise it as high as comfortably possible. Keep your leg straight but not locked at the knee.
5. Swing your left leg back behind you, maintain control, and return to the starting position.
6. Repeat this swinging motion for the desired number of repetitions, starting with 10 to 15 swings for your left leg.
7. Switch to your right leg and perform the same number of swings for balance and symmetry.

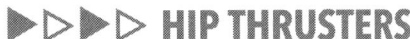 HIP THRUSTERS

Target: Glutes, quadriceps, hamstrings, and calves.
Number of sets: 3
Repetitions per set: 10 - 15 reps

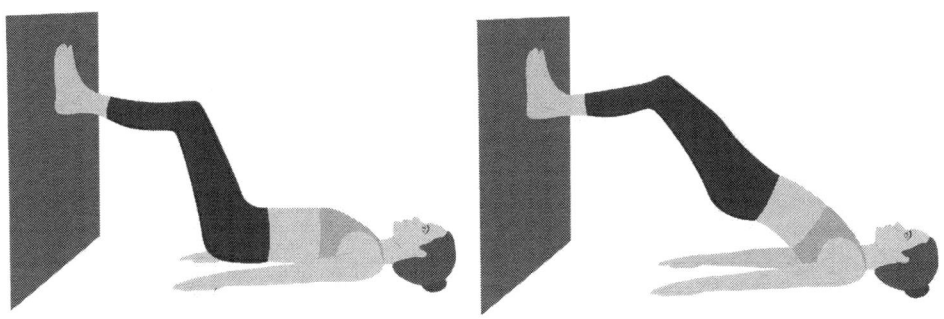

Steps

1. Lie on your back with your knees bent and your feet flat on the wall. Your feet should be hip-width apart, and your arms should be resting by your sides with your palms facing down.
2. Position yourself close to a wall so that when you lift your hips, your feet can comfortably press against the wall.
3. Engage your core muscles to maintain stability and protect your lower back.
4. Press your feet firmly into the wall, and, using your glutes and hamstrings, lift your hips off the ground. Your body should form a straight line from your shoulders to your knees at the top of the movement.
5. Hold the raised position for a moment, squeezing your glutes at the top.
6. Slowly lower your hips back down to the ground while maintaining control over the movement. Your glutes should touch the floor but not rest completely between reps to keep tension on the muscles.

▶▷▶▷ HIP THRUSTER PULSES

Target: Glutes, quadriceps, hamstrings, and calves.
Number of sets: 3
Repetitions per set: 30 - 60 seconds each set

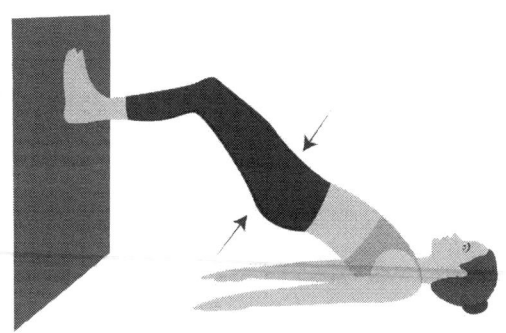

Steps

1. Lie on your back with your knees bent and your feet flat on the floor. Your feet should be hip-width apart, and your arms should be resting by your sides with your palms facing down.
2. Position yourself close to a wall so that when you lift your hips, your feet can comfortably press against the wall.
3. Engage your core muscles to maintain stability and protect your lower back.
4. Press your feet firmly into the wall, and, using your glutes and hamstrings, lift your hips off the ground. Your body should form a straight line from your shoulders to your knees at the top of the movement.
5. Hold the raised position for a moment, squeezing your glutes at the top.
6. Instead of lowering your hips all the way down, perform small, controlled pulses by lifting and lowering your hips about 1-2 inches up and down. This continuous motion targets your glutes with a pulsing movement.

▶▷▶▷ SINGLE LEG HIP THRUSTS

Target: Glutes, hip flexors, and quadriceps
Number of sets: 3
Repetitions per set: 20 to 30 reps (10 - 15 reps per leg)

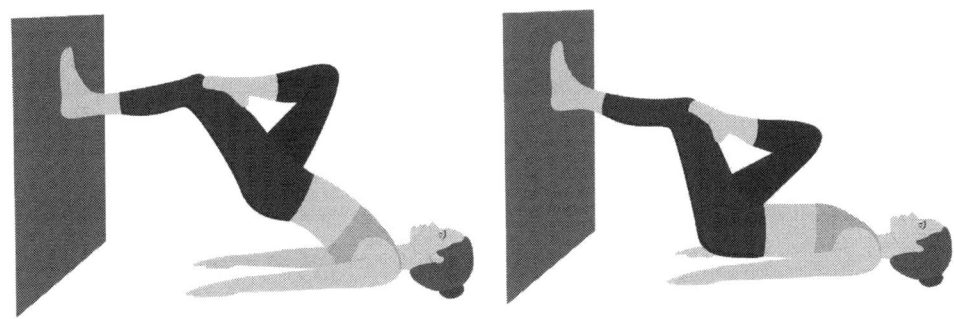

Steps

1. Lie on your back with your knees bent and your feet flat on the wall. Your feet should be hip-width apart, and your arms should be resting by your sides with your palms facing down.
2. Position yourself close to a wall so that when you lift your hips, your feet can comfortably press against the wall.
3. Engage your core muscles to maintain stability and protect your lower back.
4. Lift your right foot off the wall, extending your leg straight up toward the ceiling. Keep your left foot firmly planted on the floor. If you want it easier, you can even rest the right leg on the left, as shown in the image.
5. Press your left foot firmly into the wall, and, using your left glute and hamstring, lift your hips off the ground. Your body should form a straight line from your shoulders to your knees at the top of the movement.
6. Hold the raised position for a moment, squeezing your left glute at the top.
7. Lower your hips back down to the ground with control.
8. Repeat the lift and lower movement for the desired number of repetitions (10 to 15 reps) on your left leg.
9. After completing the repetitions on your left leg, switch to your right leg. Lower your left foot to the ground and lift your right foot up.
10. Repeat steps 4 to 8, performing 10 to 15 reps on your right leg.
11. Rest briefly between sets, and repeat for a total of 3 sets, alternating between left and right legs.

▶▷▶▷ SINGLE LEG HIP THRUSTER PULSE

Target: Glutes, hip flexors, and quadriceps
Number of sets: 3
Repetitions per set: 30 - 60 seconds each set

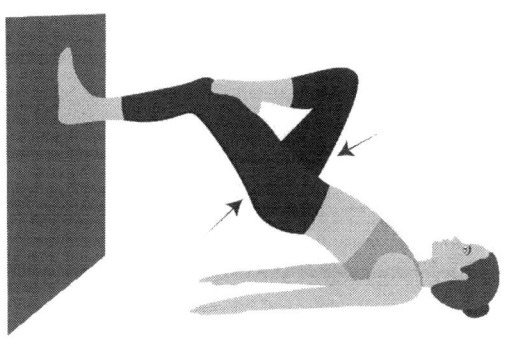

Steps

1. Lie on your back with your knees bent and your feet flat on the floor. Your feet should be hip-width apart, and your arms should be resting by your sides with your palms facing down.
2. Position yourself close to a wall so that when you lift your hips, your feet can comfortably press against the wall.
3. Engage your core muscles to maintain stability and protect your lower back.
4. Lift your right foot off the ground, extending your leg straight up toward the ceiling. Keep your left foot firmly planted on the floor.
5. For an easier modification, you can rest your right leg on your left knee, as shown in the picture.
6. Press your left foot firmly into the wall, and, using your left glute and hamstring, lift your hips off the ground. Your body should form a straight line from your shoulders to your knees at the top of the movement.
7. Hold the raised position for a moment, squeezing your left glute at the top.
8. Instead of lowering your hips all the way down, perform small, controlled pulses by lifting and lowering your hips about 1-2 inches up and down. This continuous motion targets your left glute with a pulsing movement for 30 to 60 seconds.
9. After completing the pulses on your left leg, lower your hips back down to the ground.
10. Switch to your right leg by lowering your left foot to the ground and lifting your right foot up.

▶▷▶▷ SINGLE LEG BRIDGE HOLD

Target: Glutes, hip flexors, and quadriceps
Number of sets: 3
Repetitions per set: 30 - 60 seconds each set

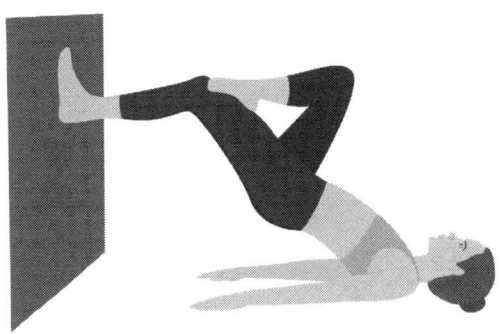

Steps

1. Lie on your back with your knees bent and your feet flat on the wall. Your feet should be hip-width apart, and your arms should be resting by your sides with your palms facing down.
2. Position yourself close to a wall so that when you lift your hips, your feet can comfortably press against the wall.
3. Engage your core muscles to maintain stability and protect your lower back.
4. Lift your right foot off the ground, extending your leg straight up toward the ceiling. Keep your left foot firmly planted on the floor.
5. If you want to make the exercise easier, you can rest your right leg on your left knee, as shown in the picture.
6. Press your left foot firmly into the wall, and, using your left glute and hamstring, lift your hips off the ground. Your body should form a straight line from your shoulders to your knees at the top of the movement.
7. Hold the raised position for 30 to 60 seconds, squeezing your left glute throughout the hold.
8. Lower your hips back down to the ground with control.
9. After completing the hold on your left leg, switch to your right leg. Lower your left foot to the ground and lift your right foot up.
10. Repeat steps 4 to 7, holding for 30 to 60 seconds on your right leg.
11. Rest briefly between sets, and repeat for a total of 3 sets, alternating between left and right legs.

CHAPTER 6. FITNESS TRACKER

Now that we have a comprehensive understanding of these workouts and how they benefit different parts of our body, it's time to create a structured plan. This plan will help us arrange these exercises effectively to maximize their benefits while avoiding overexertion and potential strain.

1. Schedule Assessment: Take a close look at your daily commitments and responsibilities. Whether you use a digital or physical calendar, record all your obligations, including work or school hours, meetings, errands, social outings, and personal dates. Ensure that you include every detail you can think of.
2. Identify Free Time: Identify periods of free time within your schedule. These could be gaps between work and social activities or extended lunch breaks. Recognize that your available time may vary from day to day, both in duration and timing.
3. Realistic Planning: Be honest with yourself about your preferences and energy levels. If you're not a morning person, scheduling an early morning workout may not be sustainable. Similarly, if you tend to feel tired after work, consider planning your workouts earlier in the day.
4. Selecting a Venue: Decide where you will exercise. You might have access to a local gym, prefer working out at home, or enjoy outdoor activities like running or walking. It's perfectly fine to mix and match these options based on your convenience and preference.
5. Exercise Selection: Choose exercises that align with your fitness goals. Start with compound movements that engage larger muscle groups before moving on to isolation exercises that target specific body parts. Your workout routine should ideally include a combination of both.
6. Gradual Progress: If you're new to exercise, avoid planning lengthy and intense workouts right from the start. Begin with shorter, 30-minute sessions every other day to allow your body to adapt and avoid burnout or injury.
7. Incorporate Rest: Understand the importance of rest in your fitness routine. Not only should you take short breaks between sets, but you should also allow sufficient rest between workouts. Muscles need time to recover and grow, so aim for 24 to 48 hours of rest between exercise sessions.
8. Tolerance Building: Recognize that varying the number of repetitions (reps) can yield different results. Focus on building endurance and muscle memory with 2-3 sets of 10-15 reps using light weights. As you progress, adjust your routine to include heavier weights and lower reps for strength and size gains.

Crafting an effective exercise plan is a systematic process that begins with a clear goal in mind. Whether you aim to build strength, enhance cardiovascular fitness, or improve flexibility, specificity is key. Tailor your workout routine to align with your objectives, incorporating exercises that address your target muscle groups or skills.

Consistency is paramount for sustainable progress, so establish a workout frequency that suits your lifestyle. For those training three times a week or less, total-body workouts can be highly effective. On the other hand, individuals planning four or more weekly sessions should diversify their routines, focusing on movement types rather than specific body parts.

Remember that the body adapts over time, so periodic change is essential to avoid plateauing. Regularly update your routine by altering equipment, set and rep schemes, or exercise variations while maintaining a dedicated day of rest each week. By following these steps and staying open to adaptation, you can create a workout plan that not only keeps you engaged but also maximizes your fitness gains.

Fitness Plans for the Month

Here are examples of a couple of plans that you could use with the exercises prescribed in the books. The first plan is one that segregates the workouts based on the days.

DAILY FITNESS ROUTINE (WEEK 1)

DAY 1	DAY 2	DAY 3	DAY 4	DAY 5	DAY 6	DAY 7
Abs: Bridge Raises (3 sets of 10-15 reps)	Abs: Crunches (3 sets of 10-15 reps)	Rest or Light Stretching	Abs: Crunch Twister (3 sets of 10-15 reps)	Abs: Bridge Knee to Chest Exercise (3 sets of 10-15 reps)	Abs: One-Leg Bridge Raise (3 sets of 10-15 reps per leg)	Rest or Light Stretching
Back Posture: Wall Push-Ups (3 sets of 10-15 reps)	Back Posture: One Arm Wall Push-Ups (3 sets of 10-15 reps per arm)	Rest or Light Stretching	Back Posture: Plank Shoulder Taps (3 sets of 10-15 reps per arm)	Back Posture: Elbow to Plank (3 sets of 10-15 reps)	Back Posture: Wall Angels (3 sets of 10-15 reps)	Rest or Light Stretching
Buttocks: Kick Backs (3 sets of 10-15 reps per leg)	Buttocks: Split Squats (3 sets of 10-15 reps per leg)	Rest or Light Stretching	Buttocks: Wall Squats (3 sets of 10-15 reps)	Buttocks: Wall Sit (Wall Squat Hold) (3 sets of 30-60 seconds)	Buttocks: Forward Wall Squat (3 sets of 10-15 reps)	Rest or Light Stretching

WEEK 2, 3, AND 4:

- Continue with a similar pattern, progressively increasing repetitions or sets as you feel more comfortable.
- Include warm-up and cool-down routines.
- Prioritize proper form and technique over the number of repetitions.
- Listen to your body and rest when needed.
- Consider incorporating cardiovascular exercises on rest days.
- Maintain a balanced diet, hydration, and adequate sleep.
- Adjust intensity and frequency as needed to align with your fitness goals.
- Consult a fitness professional for personalized guidance and modifications if required.

FITNESS ROUTINE BASED ON WORKOUTS

DAY	ABS	BACK POSTURE	BUTTOCKS
1	Bridge Raises (3 sets of 10-15 reps)	Wall Push-Ups (3 sets of 10-15 reps)	Kick Backs (3 sets of 10-15 reps per leg)
2	Crunches (3 sets of 10-15 reps)	One Arm Wall Push-Ups (3 sets of 10-15 reps per arm)	Split Squats (3 sets of 10-15 reps per leg)
3	Rest or Light Stretching	Plank Shoulder Taps (3 sets of 10-15 reps per arm)	Rest or Light Stretching
4	Crunch Twister (3 sets of 10-15 reps)	Elbow to Plank (3 sets of 10-15 reps)	Wall Squats (3 sets of 10-15 reps)
5	Bridge Knee to Chest Exercise (3 sets of 10-15 reps)	Wall Angels (3 sets of 10-15 reps)	Wall Sit (Wall Squat Hold) (3 sets of 30-60 seconds)
6	One-Leg Bridge Raise (3 sets of 10-15 reps per leg)	Chest Opener (3 sets of 10-15 reps)	Forward Wall Squat (3 sets of 10-15 reps)
7	Rest or Light Stretching	Shoulder Press (3 sets of 10-15 reps)	Rest or Light Stretching
8	Crunches (3 sets of 10-15 reps)	Isometric Pulls (3 sets of 10-15 reps)	Hip Thrusters (3 sets of 10-15 reps)
9	Knee to Chest (3 sets of 10-15 reps)	Diamond Push Ups (3 sets of 10-15 reps)	Hip Thruster Pulses (3 sets of 30-60 seconds)
10	Rest or Light Stretching	Wall Push-Ups (3 sets of 10-15 reps)	Rest or Light Stretching
11	One-Leg Bridge Raise (3 sets of 10-15 reps per leg)	One Arm Wall Push-Ups (3 sets of 10-15 reps per arm)	Lateral Leg Swings (3 sets of 10-15 reps per leg)
12	Toe Reaches (3 sets of 10-15 reps)	Plank Shoulder Taps (3 sets of 10-15 reps per arm)	Forward Leg Swings (3 sets of 10-15 reps per leg)
13	3-Second Bear Crawl (3 sets of 10-15 reps)	Elbow to Plank (3 sets of 10-15 reps)	Hip Thrusters (3 sets of 10-15 reps)
14	Rest or Light Stretching	Wall Angels (3 sets of 10-15 reps)	Rest or Light Stretching

15	Crunch Twister (3 sets of 10-15 reps)	Chest Opener (3 sets of 10-15 reps)	Single Leg Hip Thrusts (3 sets of 10-15 reps per leg)
16	Bridge Knee to Chest Exercise (3 sets of 10-15 reps)	Shoulder Press (3 sets of 10-15 reps)	Single Leg Hip Thruster Pulses (3 sets of 30-60 seconds per leg)
17	Rest or Light Stretching	Leg Curls (3 sets of 10-15 reps)	Rest or Light Stretching
18	One-Leg Bridge Raise (3 sets of 10-15 reps per leg)	Toe Touches (3 sets of 10-15 reps)	Hip Thrusters (3 sets of 10-15 reps)
19	Crunches (3 sets of 10-15 reps)	Isometric Pulls (3 sets of 10-15 reps)	Hip Thruster Pulses (3 sets of 30-60 seconds)
20	V-Sit Ups (3 sets of 10-15 reps)	Wall Push-Ups (3 sets of 10-15 reps)	Lateral Leg Swings (3 sets of 10-15 reps per leg)
21	Rest or Light Stretching	Plank Shoulder Taps (3 sets of 10-15 reps per arm)	Forward Leg Swings (3 sets of 10-15 reps per leg)
22	Bridge Raises (3 sets of 10-15 reps)	Wall Push-Ups (3 sets of 10-15 reps)	Kick Backs (3 sets of 10-15 reps per leg)
23	Crunches (3 sets of 10-15 reps)	One Arm Wall Push-Ups (3 sets of 10-15 reps per arm)	Split Squats (3 sets of 10-15 reps per leg)
24	Rest or Light Stretching	Plank Shoulder Taps (3 sets of 10-15 reps per arm)	Rest or Light Stretching
25	Crunch Twister (3 sets of 10-15 reps)	Elbow to Plank (3 sets of 10-15 reps)	Wall Squats (3 sets of 10-15 reps)
26	Bridge Knee to Chest Exercise (3 sets of 10-15 reps)	Wall Angels (3 sets of 10-15 reps)	Wall Sit (Wall Squat Hold) (3 sets of 30-60 seconds)
27	One-Leg Bridge Raise (3 sets of 10-15 reps per leg)	Chest Opener (3 sets of 10-15 reps)	Forward Wall Squat (3 sets of 10-15 reps)
28	Rest or Light Stretching	Shoulder Press (3 sets of 10-15 reps)	Rest or Light Stretching
29	Crunches (3 sets of 10-15 reps)	Isometric Pulls (3 sets of 10-15 reps)	Hip Thrusters (3 sets of 10-15 reps)
30	Knee to Chest (3 sets of 10-15 reps)	Diamond Push Ups (3 sets of 10-15 reps)	Hip Thruster Pulses (3 sets of 30-60 seconds)

Feel free to adjust the repetitions, sets, or exercises based on your fitness level and preferences.

Remember to incorporate rest days and stay hydrated throughout your fitness journey.

CHAPTER 7. EATING THE RIGHT NUTRITION

To fully benefit from Pilates as a mind and body fitness regimen, it's essential to consider the types of foods that keep you feeling balanced and energized.

Pre-Pilates Session

Before a Pilates session, it's advisable to avoid foods that might cause gas or an upset stomach. Opt for complex carbohydrates and lean proteins, along with a bit of healthy fat, as they provide sustained energy compared to simple carbs or sugary snacks.

Here are some suggestions for a light pre-Pilates meal:

- A protein shake with fruit can be a convenient choice, and you can adjust the portion size to your preference.
- Peanut butter on whole-grain bread offers a quick source of complex carbohydrates and protein.
- Yogurt with fruit or a small serving of oatmeal can provide essential carbohydrates.

Given the emphasis on abdominal muscles in Pilates, it's crucial to allow ample time for digestion before your session. Aim for a light meal or snack, such as a banana or a smoothie that provides carbohydrates for energy.

Nutrition experts recommend waiting two to three hours after eating before exercising. If you've skipped breakfast or it's been an extended period since your last meal, consider having a light snack to ensure you have sufficient energy during your workout.

Post-Pilates Session

After a Pilates session, your body requires the necessary nutrients to repair and strengthen muscles while replenishing energy stores. Consider consuming a protein-rich green smoothie or a light snack containing lean protein like fish or chicken, coupled with carbohydrates from whole grains.

Your dietary choices between workouts will depend on whether your goal is weight loss. Regardless, it's essential to eat in a way that suits your body. While Pilates can complement cardiovascular exercise in a weight loss plan, it's crucial to remember that exercise alone is unlikely to lead to significant weight loss. Caloric intake reduction is often necessary.

Engaging in Pilates can encourage you to prioritize nutritious foods while minimizing empty calories, which can have positive health effects, whether your goal is weight loss or not. Opt for a diet aligned with the current U.S. Dietary Guidelines.

Pilates Hydration Advice

Pilates is generally considered to be a light-to-moderate-intensity exercise and typically doesn't necessitate specialized sports drinks. However, proper hydration is crucial. Water remains an excellent choice.

Ensure you drink an 8-ounce glass of water around 30 minutes before your class, allowing your body time to eliminate excess fluids and start adequately hydrated. Keep a water bottle handy during your session to sip when needed. After your workout, rehydrate with at least 16 ounces of water within 30 minutes.

Staying well-hydrated supports your overall health and enhances your Pilates experience.

Bonus Recipes

Here are 7 of my favorite recipes I would like to share with you that are not just balanced meals but also work incredibly well with Pilates.

▶▷▶▷ SPAGHETTI SEAFOOD CARBONARA

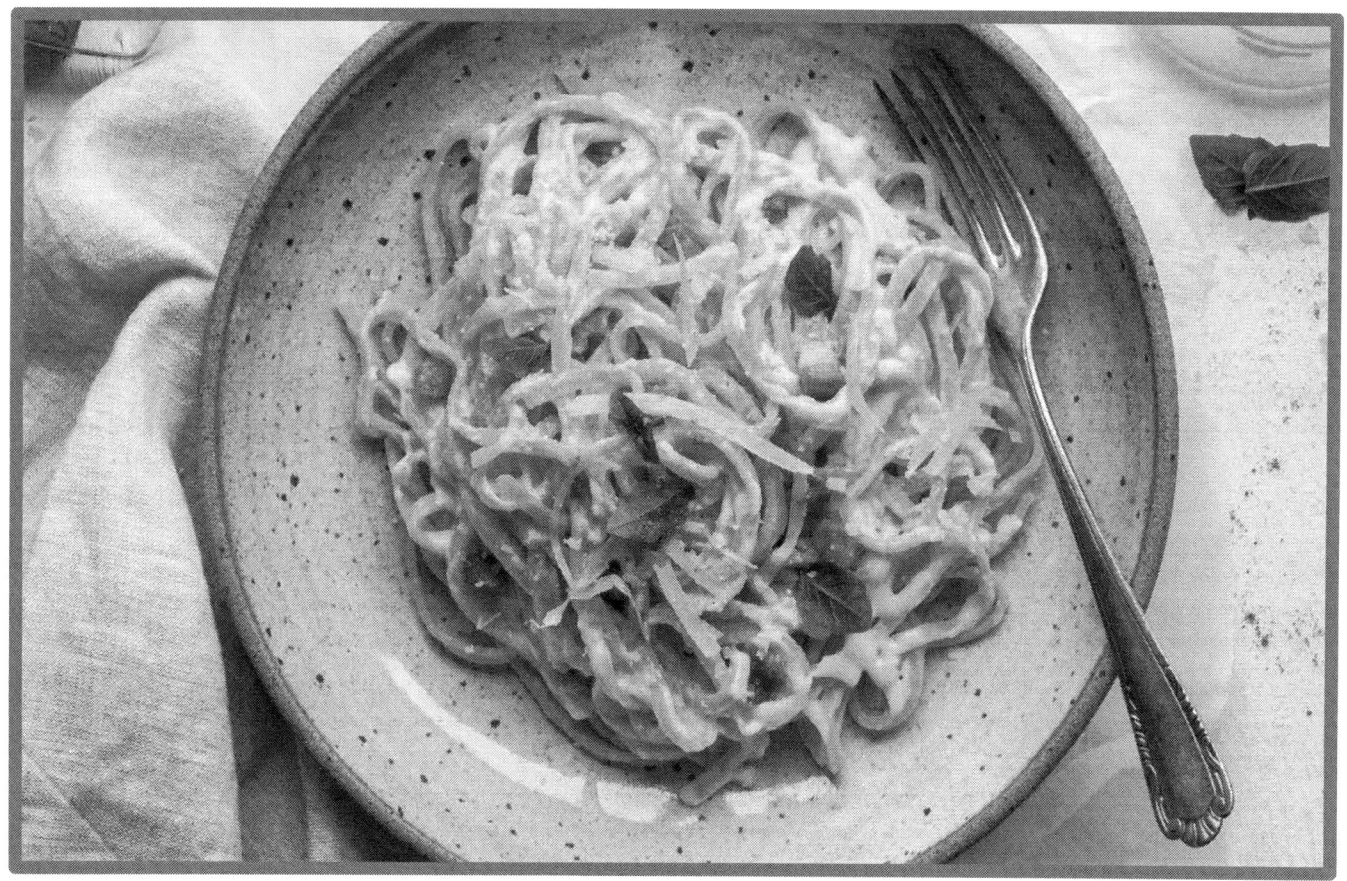

Preparation Time: 15 minutes
Cooking Time: 15 minutes
Total Time: 30 minutes
Servings: 4
Nutritional Value: 475 calories, 21 g protein, 32 g carbs, 30 g fat

Ingredients:

- 8 ounces spaghetti
- 4 slices of bacon, chopped
- 1 small onion, finely chopped
- 2 cloves garlic, minced

- 1 cup mixed seafood (shrimp, mussels, and calamari), cleaned and chopped
- 2 large eggs
- 1/2 cup grated Parmesan cheese
- 1/4 cup heavy cream
- Salt and black pepper to taste
- Fresh parsley, chopped, for garnish

Prep Instructions

1. Prepare your spaghetti by cooking it according to the package instructions until it's al dente.
2. Drain and set aside.
3. In a large skillet, cook the chopped bacon over medium heat until crispy–about 5 minutes.
4. Remove the bacon from the skillet, leaving the bacon drippings.
5. In the same skillet, add the onion and minced garlic.
6. Sauté until they become translucent, about 2 minutes.
7. Add the mixed seafood to the skillet with the sautéed onions and garlic.
8. Cook for another 3-4 minutes until the seafood is cooked through and opaque.
9. Remove from heat.

Cooking Method

1. In a mixing bowl, whisk together the eggs, grated Parmesan cheese, heavy cream, and a pinch of black pepper.
2. Mix until well combined.
3. Return the cooked spaghetti to the pot or a large bowl.
4. Add the crispy bacon pieces and toss them together.
5. Quickly pour the egg and cheese mixture over the hot pasta and bacon.
6. Toss vigorously to coat the pasta evenly–the heat from the pasta will cook the eggs and create a creamy sauce.
7. Gently fold the cooked mixed seafood, onions, and garlic into the pasta and egg mixture.
8. Taste the pasta and season with salt and additional black pepper as needed–be cautious with salt since the bacon and Parmesan are already salty.
9. Garnish your seafood carbonara with chopped fresh parsley.
10. Serve hot, and enjoy your homemade Spaghetti Seafood Carbonara!

▶▷▶▷ ZUCCHINI FRITTERS RECIPE

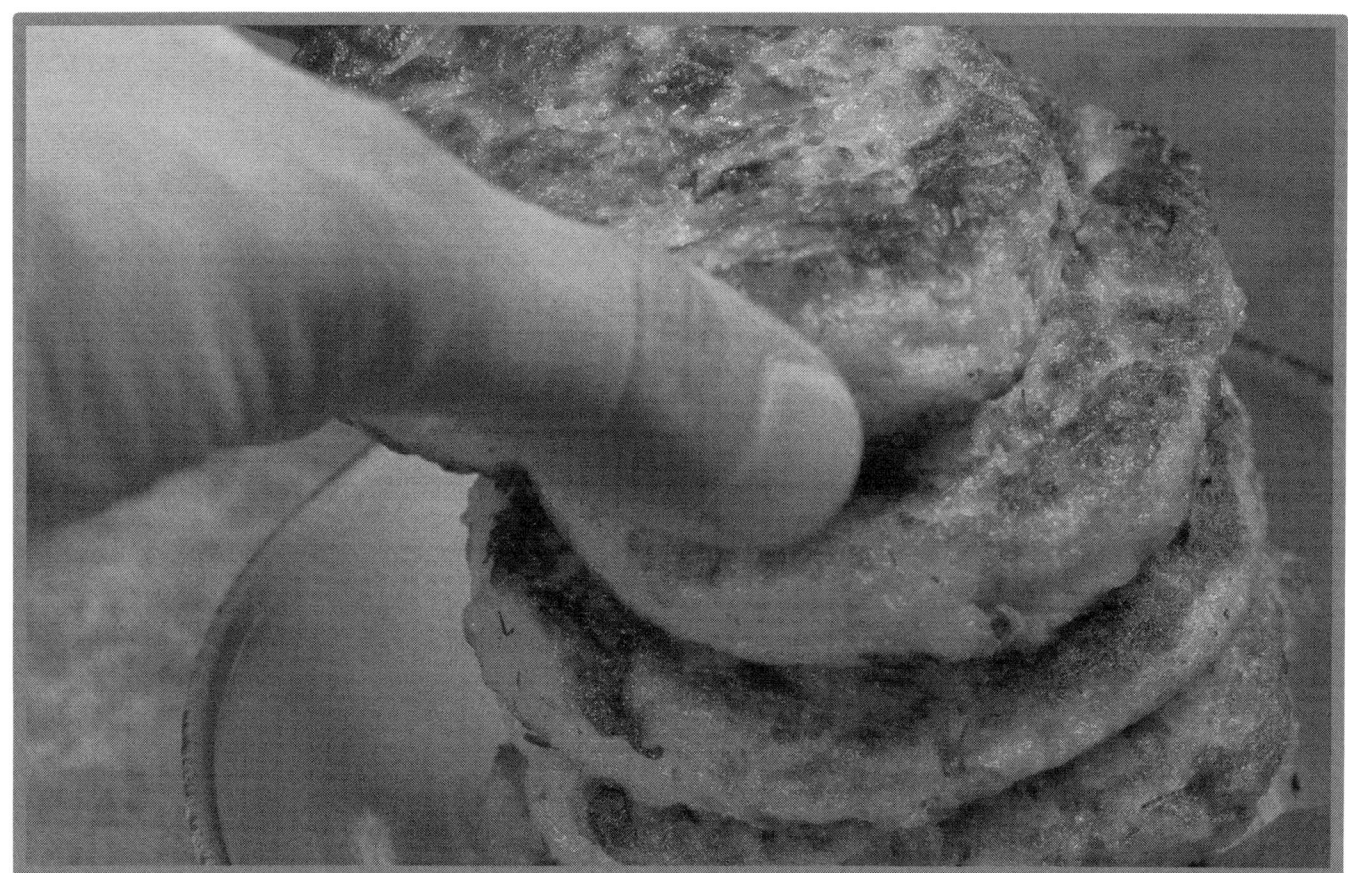

Preparation Time: 15 minutes
Cooking Time: 15 minutes
Total Time: 30 minutes
Servings: 4
Nutritional Value: 175 calories, 8g fat, 19g carbs, 8g protein

Ingredients:

- 2 medium-sized zucchini
- 1 teaspoon salt
- 1/2 cup all-purpose flour
- 1/4 cup grated Parmesan cheese
- 1/4 cup shredded mozzarella cheese
- 2 cloves garlic, minced
- 1 large egg, beaten
- 2 tablespoons fresh basil leaves, chopped
- 1/2 teaspoon black pepper

- Olive oil for frying

Prep Instructions:

1. Wash the zucchini.
2. Using a grater or food processor, grate the zucchini.
3. Place the grated zucchini in a colander and sprinkle with 1 teaspoon of salt.
4. Allow it to sit for about 10 minutes to draw out excess moisture.
5. Use your hands to squeeze out as much liquid as possible from the grated zucchini.
6. Place the squeezed zucchini in a clean kitchen towel and pat out any remaining moisture.
7. In a large mixing bowl, combine the grated zucchini, all-purpose flour, grated Parmesan cheese, shredded mozzarella cheese, minced garlic, beaten egg, chopped fresh basil, and black pepper.
8. Mix everything together until you have a thick batter.

Cooking Method

1. Heat a large skillet or frying pan over medium-high heat and add enough olive oil to cover the bottom of the pan.
2. Carefully scoop spoonfuls of the zucchini batter into the skillet, flattening them slightly with the back of the spoon.
3. Ensure you don't overcrowd the pan, and leave some space between each fritter.
4. Cook the fritters for about 2-3 minutes on each side, or until they are golden brown and crispy.
5. Use a spatula to flip them over and cook for another 2-3 minutes.
6. Transfer the cooked zucchini fritters to a plate lined with paper towels to remove excess oil.
7. Serve the zucchini fritters hot, garnished with additional fresh basil if desired.
8. They can be enjoyed on their own or with a dipping sauce of your choice, such as tzatziki or marinara.

▶▷▶▷ MEXICAN EGGS WITH POTATO HASH

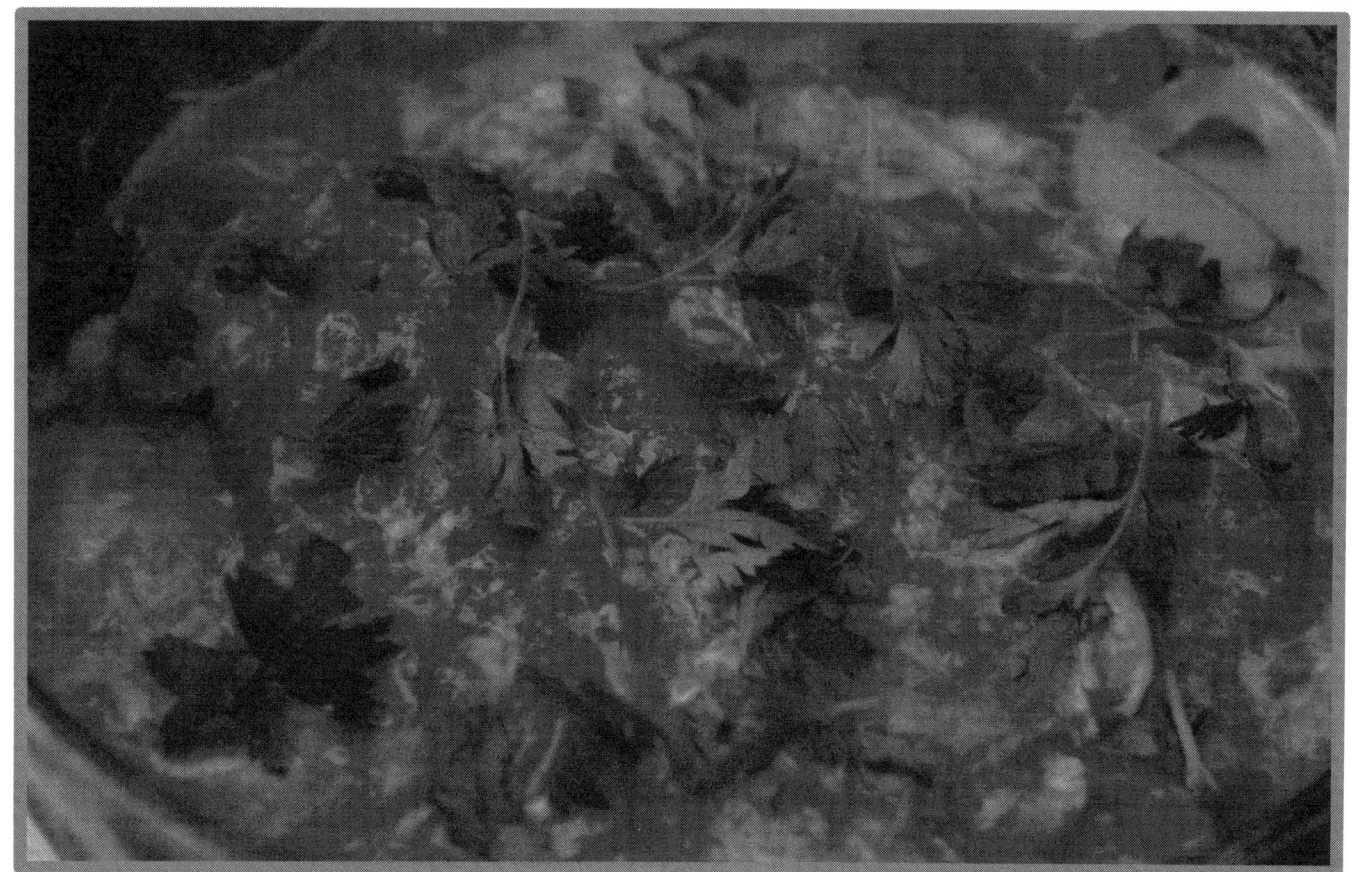

Preparation Time: 15 minutes
Cooking Time: 20 minutes
Total Time: 35 minutes
Servings: 4
Nutritional Value: 420 calories, 22g protein, 25g carbs, 27g fat

Ingredients:

For the Beef:

- 1 tablespoon oil
- 1 onion, finely chopped
- Pinch of salt
- 300g ground beef
- 2 tablespoons chipotle sauce
- 400g can diced tomatoes
- 2 tablespoons chopped fresh coriander
- Freshly ground black pepper, to taste

For the Potato Hash:

- 2 large potatoes, peeled and coarsely grated
- 2 tablespoons melted butter
- Salt and freshly ground black pepper, to taste
- 2 tablespoons oil (for frying)

For the Eggs:

- 4 large eggs

To Garnish:

- Sliced chili (adjust to your spice preference)
- Extra fresh coriander leaves

Prep Instructions:

Prepare the Beef:

1. Heat 1 tablespoon of oil in a large frypan with a lid over medium-high heat.
2. Add finely chopped onion and a pinch of salt.
3. Cook, stirring occasionally, for 3-4 minutes or until the onion is soft.
4. Add the ground beef and cook, breaking it apart with a spoon, for about 5 minutes or until browned.
5. Stir in the chipotle sauce, diced tomatoes, and chopped fresh coriander.
6. Season with freshly ground black pepper.
7. Reduce the heat to medium and let it simmer for a further 5-6 minutes or until slightly thickened.

Prepare the Potato Hash:

1. Place the coarsely grated potato in a clean tea towel and squeeze it to remove excess water.
2. Transfer the squeezed potato to a bowl and add the melted butter.
3. Season the potato mixture with salt and freshly ground black pepper, then stir to combine.
4. Heat 1 tablespoon of oil in a separate frypan over medium heat.
5. Using a 1/3 cup (80ml) measuring cup, place 4 mounds of potato in the pan, flatten them with a spoon.
6. Flip the hash once brown, about 3-4 minutes.

7. Cook for 3-4 minutes on each side until they are golden and cooked through.
8. Repeat this process with the remaining 1 tablespoon of oil and the potato mixture.

Cook the Eggs:

1. Using a spoon, make 4 indents in the beef mixture.
2. Crack one egg into each indent.
3. Cover the pan and cook for 7 minutes or until the egg whites are cooked and the yolks are still slightly runny.

Serve:

- Garnish the Mexican eggs with sliced chili and extra fresh coriander leaves.
- Serve alongside the crispy potato hash.

▶▷▶▷ LEMON CHICKEN

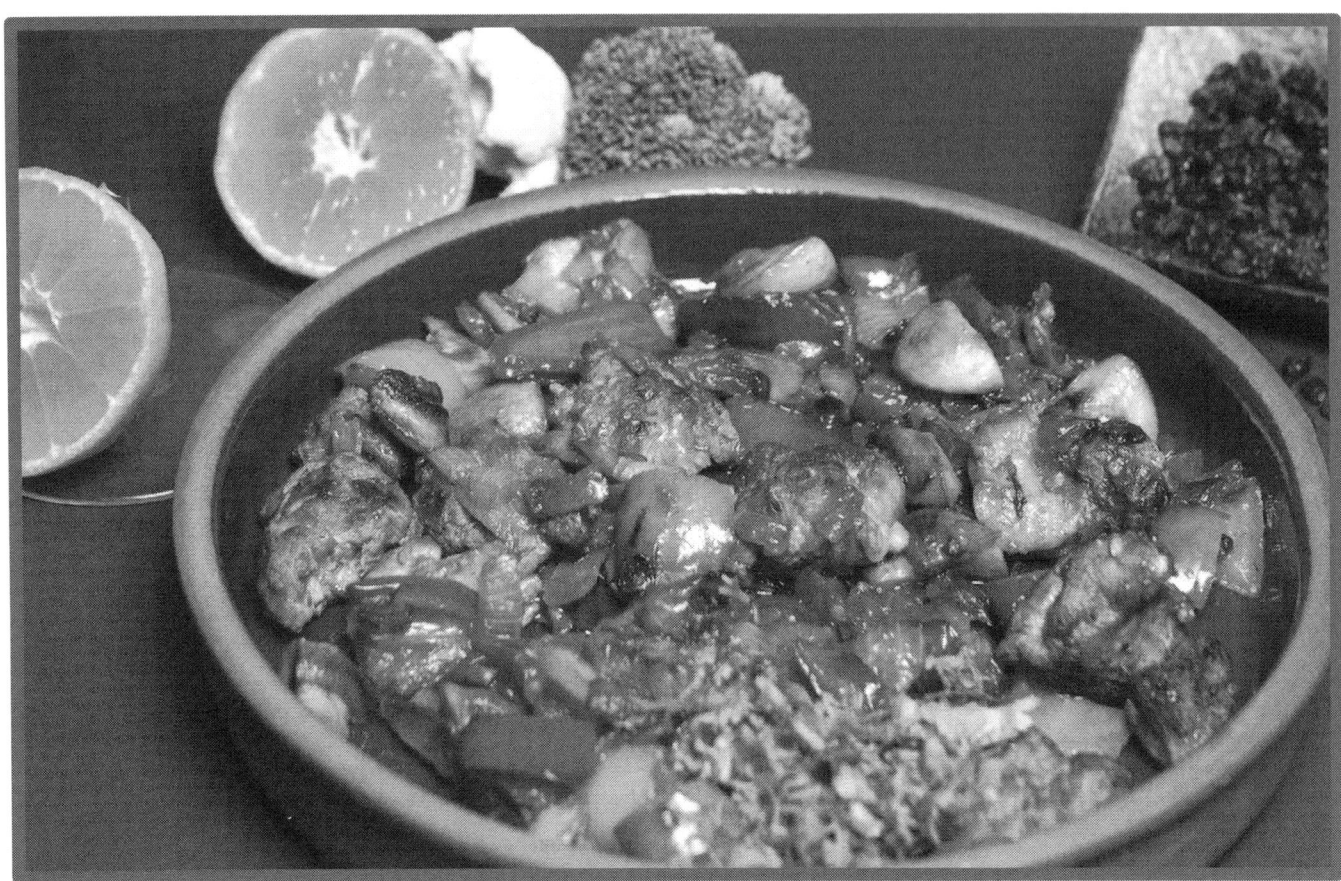

Preparation Time: 10 minutes
Cooking Time: 10 minutes
Total Time: 20 minutes
Serves: 4
Nutritional Value: 250-300 calories, 20-25 g protein, 15 g carbs, 12 g fat

Ingredients:

- 2 tablespoons oil of your choice
- 1 cup carrots, thinly sliced
- 2 cups broccoli florets
- 3 tablespoons spring onions, roughly chopped
- 4 cloves fresh garlic, minced
- 1 pound boneless, skinless chicken breasts, cubed
- ¼ cup chicken broth, low sodium if preferred
- ¼ soya sauce, low sodium if preferred
- 3 tablespoons honey

- 2 tablespoons lemon juice, freshly squeezed or store bought
- ¼ teaspoon capsicum
- 2 teaspoons cornstarch
- Salt and pepper to taste

Prep Instructions:

1. In a small bowl, mix the cornflour, soy sauce, and lemon juice until well combined.
2. Heat the oil in a large frying pan or wok over high heat.
3. Add the chicken, capsicum, carrot, and broccoli to the hot pan.
4. Stir-fry for 2–3 minutes, or until the chicken is lightly browned, and the vegetables are beginning to soften.

Cooking Method:

1. Pour the prepared lemon and soy mixture into the pan with the chicken and vegetables.
2. Add the chicken stock and spring onions to the pan.
3. Bring the mixture to a simmer
4. Reduce the heat.
5. Cook for an additional 2 minutes, or until the sauce is slightly thickened, and the chicken is cooked through, stirring continuously.
6. Sprinkle the dish with grated lemon zest for an extra burst of flavor.
7. Serve your delicious lemon chicken with rice and enjoy!

▶▷▶▷ GARLIC PORK FRIED RICE

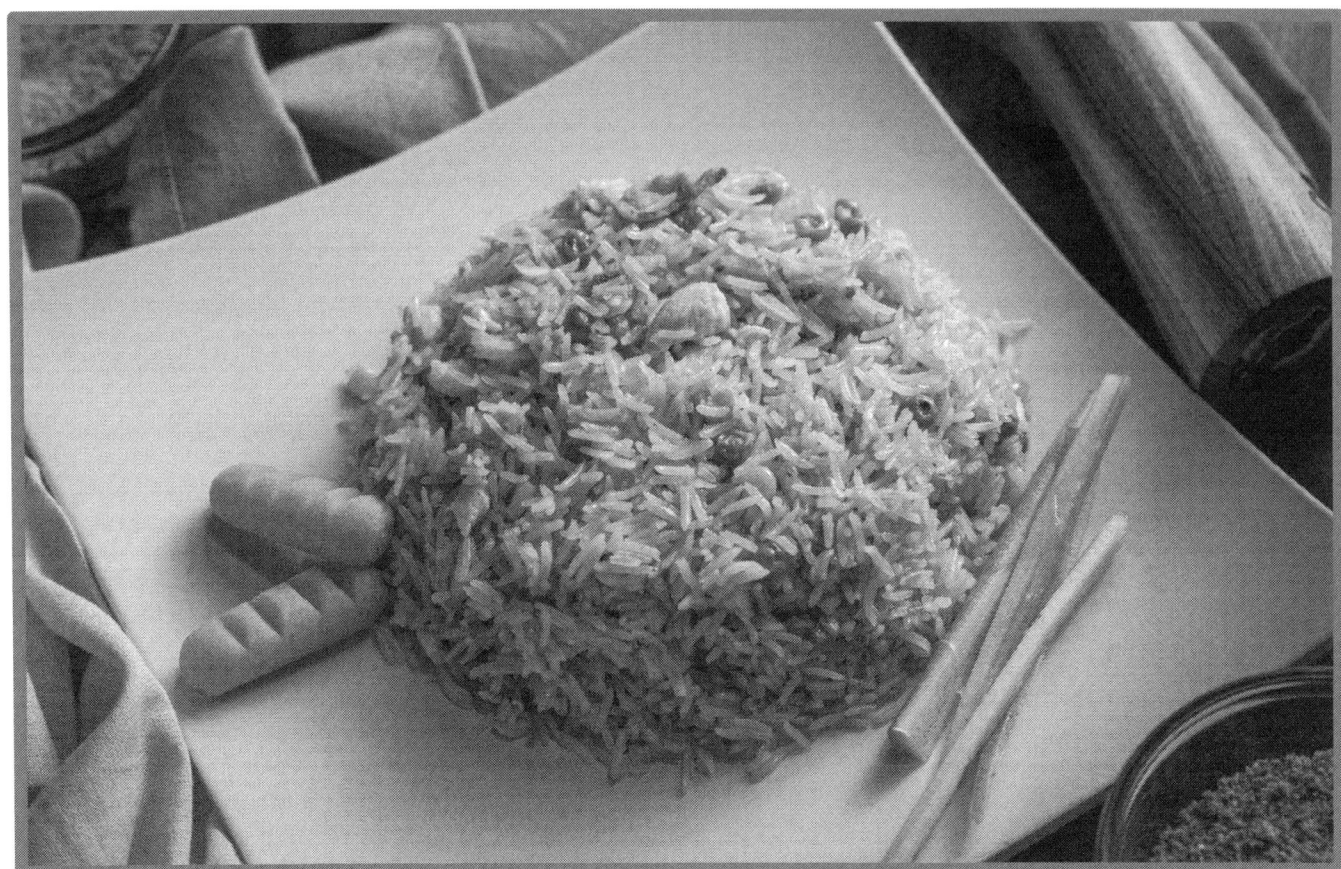

Preparation Time: 15 minutes
Cooking Time: 15 minutes
Total Time: 30 minutes
Serves: 4
Nutritional Value: 380 calories, 15g protein, 42g carbs, 17g fat

Ingredients:

- 2 cups cooked rice (preferably chilled)
- 250g pork, thinly sliced
- 4 cloves garlic, minced
- 1 cup mixed vegetables (peas, carrots, corn)
- 2 eggs, beaten
- 2 tablespoons soy sauce
- 1 tablespoon oyster sauce
- 1/2 teaspoon sesame oil
- Salt and pepper to taste

- 2 tablespoons cooking oil
- Green onions, chopped, for garnish

Prep Instructions:
1. Cook the rice according to package instructions.
2. Cool the rice in the refrigerator–chilled rice works best for fried rice.
3. Thinly slice the pork.
4. Mince the garlic.
5. Beat the eggs in a bowl.
6. Measure out the soy sauce, oyster sauce, and sesame oil.
7. Chop the green onions for garnish.

Cooking Method
1. Heat 1 tablespoon of cooking oil in a large wok or frying pan over medium-high heat.
2. Add the minced garlic and sauté for about 30 seconds until fragrant.
3. Add the sliced pork and stir-fry until it turns brown and is cooked through, about 3-4 minutes.
4. Remove the pork from the pan and set it aside.
5. In the same pan, add the remaining 1 tablespoon of cooking oil.
6. Add the mixed vegetables and stir-fry for 2-3 minutes until they start to soften.
7. Push the vegetables to one side of the pan and pour the beaten eggs into the other side.
8. Scramble the eggs until they are fully cooked.
9. Add the cooked pork back into the pan with the scrambled eggs and vegetables.
10. Add the chilled cooked rice to the pan and stir-fry everything together.
11. Pour the soy sauce, oyster sauce, and sesame oil over the fried rice.
12. Season with salt and pepper to taste.
13. Continue to stir-fry for another 3-4 minutes, ensuring the rice is evenly coated with the sauces.
14. Transfer the garlic pork fried rice to serving plates.

▶▷▶▷ LAMB CHOPS AND ROASTED POTATOES

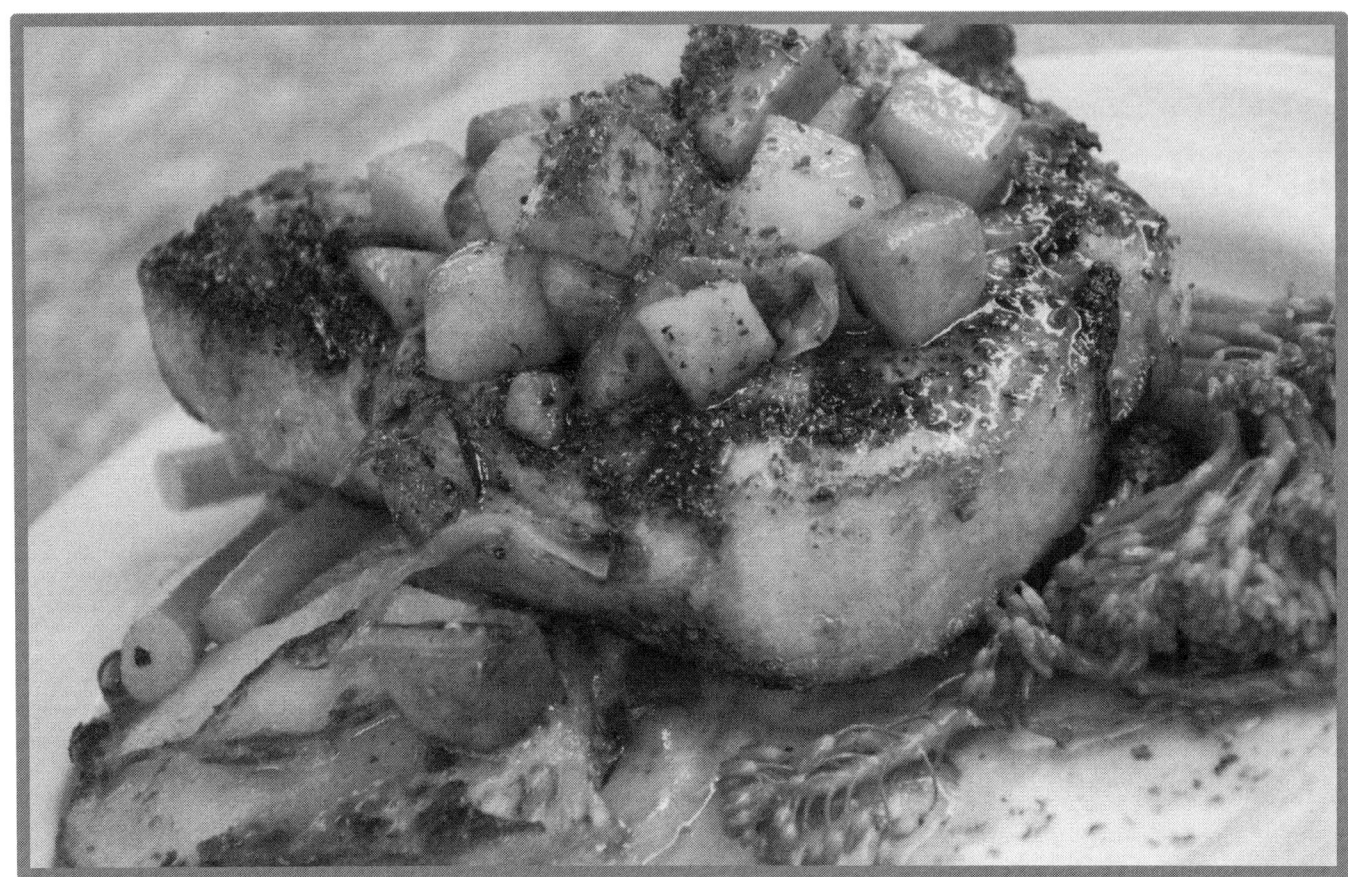

Preparation Time: 15 minutes
Cooking Time: 40 minutes
Total Time: 55 minutes
Serves: 4
Nutritional Value: 290 calories, 25g protein, 25g carbs, 20g fat

Ingredients:

- 4 lamb chops
- 2 tablespoons olive oil
- 2 cloves garlic, minced
- 1 teaspoon fresh rosemary, chopped
- Salt and black pepper to taste
- 4 large potatoes, peeled and cut into chunks
- 2 tablespoons olive oil
- 1 teaspoon dried oregano
- 1 teaspoon dried thyme

- Salt and black pepper to taste

Prep Instructions:

1. In a small bowl, combine the minced garlic, chopped rosemary, olive oil, salt, and black pepper.
2. Brush the mixture evenly over both sides of the lamb chops and let them marinate for at least 15 minutes at room temperature.
3. Preheat your oven to 425°F (220°C).
4. In a large mixing bowl, toss the potato chunks with olive oil, dried oregano, dried thyme, salt, and black pepper until they are well coated.

Cooking Method

For the Lamb Chops:

1. Preheat a grill or grill pan over medium-high heat.
2. Grill the lamb chops for about 4-5 minutes per side for medium-rare, adjusting the time for your preferred level of doneness.
3. Remove the lamb chops from the grill and let them rest for a few minutes before serving.
4. Spread the seasoned potato chunks in a single layer on a baking sheet.
5. Roast your vegetables in the oven for approximately 25-30 minutes or until they are golden brown and tender when pierced with a fork.
6. Serve the grilled lamb chops alongside the roasted potatoes for a delicious and satisfying meal.

▶▷▶▷ CHICKPEA SALAD

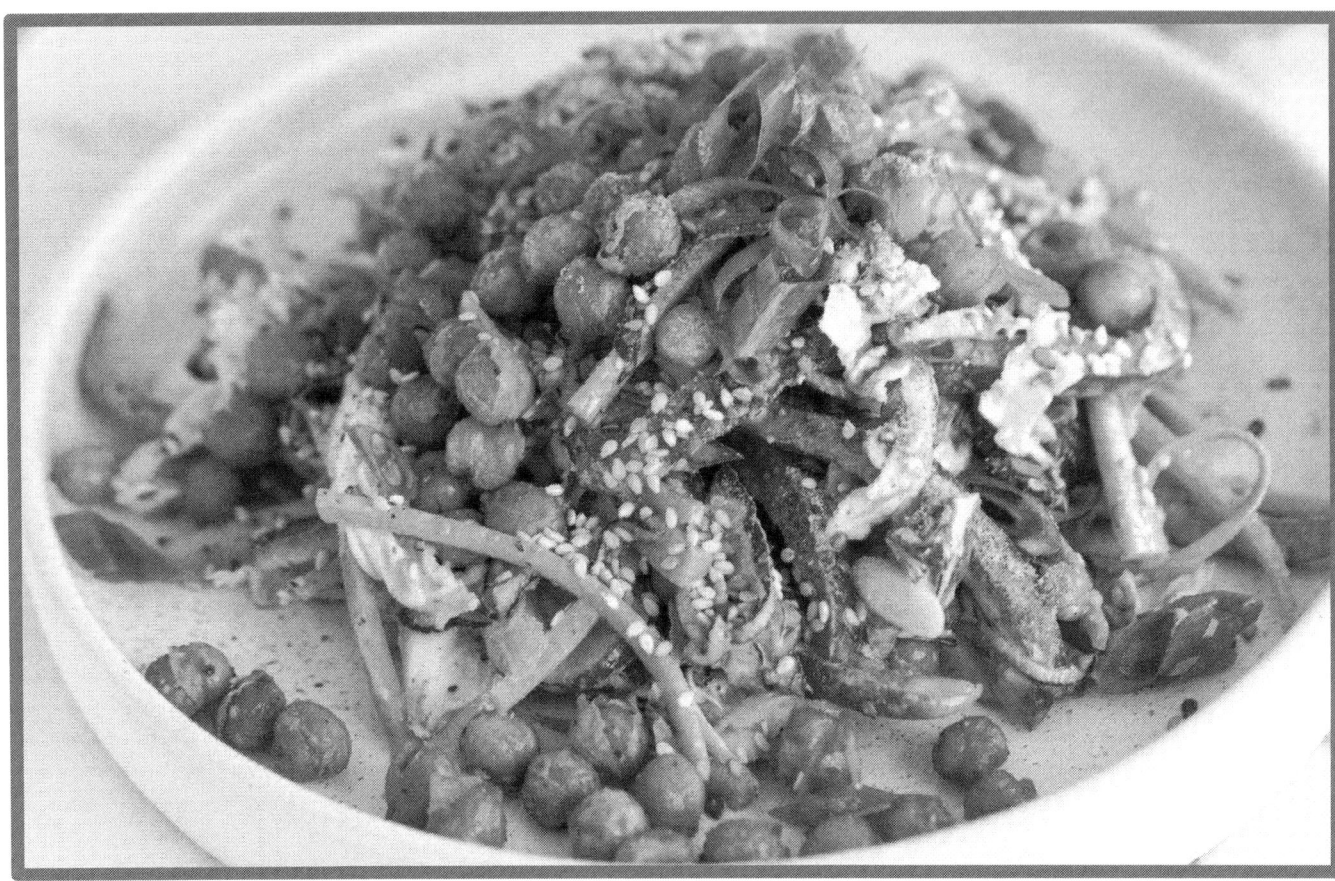

Preparation Time: 15 minutes
Total Time: 15 minutes
Serves: 4-6
Nutritional Value: 300 calories, 12 g protein, 35 g carbs, 15 g fat

Ingredients:

- 2 cans (15 ounces each) chickpeas, drained and rinsed
- 1 cucumber, diced
- 1 cup cherry tomatoes, halved
- 1/2 red onion, finely chopped
- 1/2 cup fresh parsley, chopped
- 1/4 cup fresh mint leaves, chopped
- 1/3 cup feta cheese, crumbled
- 1/4 cup Kalamata olives, pitted and sliced
- Juice of 1 lemon
- 3 tablespoons extra-virgin olive oil

- 2 cloves garlic, minced
- 1 teaspoon ground cumin
- Salt and pepper to taste

Cooking Method:

1. In a large salad bowl, combine the drained and rinsed chickpeas, diced cucumber, halved cherry tomatoes, finely chopped red onion, fresh parsley, and fresh mint leaves.
2. In a small bowl, whisk together the lemon juice, extra-virgin olive oil, minced garlic, ground cumin, salt, and pepper to create the dressing.
3. Drizzle the dressing over the salad ingredients in a large bowl.
4. Toss the salad gently to ensure that the dressing coats all the ingredients evenly.
5. Add the crumbled feta cheese and sliced Kalamata olives to the salad.
6. Taste the salad and adjust the seasoning with additional salt, pepper, or lemon juice if desired.
7. Serve immediately or refrigerate it for a few hours to allow the flavors to meld together before serving.

CONCLUSION

As we conclude this journey into the world of Wall Pilates for women, it's crucial to leave you with some key insights to carry forward:

- **Breathing Matters:** Throughout your Wall Pilates practice, remember the importance of controlled and steady breathing. Proper breathing not only enhances blood circulation but also detoxifies your body and activates muscle groups, contributing to a more effective workout.
- **Embrace Post-Workout Soreness:** Don't be surprised if you experience soreness after a Wall Pilates session. Despite its low-impact nature, Wall Pilates engages various muscle groups intensely. Post-workout soreness is a sign that your body is getting stronger and more toned.
- **Dress for Success:** When it comes to attire, opt for form-fitting clothes during your Wall Pilates sessions. This choice allows you to monitor your movements clearly and prevents any wardrobe mishaps with the equipment, ensuring a smoother and more focused workout.
- **Listen to Your Body:** In Wall Pilates, the mantra is "no pain, no gain" should be replaced with "if there's pain, there's no gain." Always tune in to your body's signals and respect its limits. Wall Pilates is a deliberate and gradual practice; rushing through it won't yield better results. Taking your time during each exercise can enhance the challenge and effectiveness.
- **Workout Frequency:** The most effective exercise routine is the one you commit to. Whether you integrate Wall Pilates into your schedule once a week or more frequently, choose a frequency that aligns with your practicality, convenience, and sustainability.
- **Evidence-Based Benefits:** Research suggests that incorporating a minimum of two 60-minute Wall Pilates sessions per week can deliver significant benefits. These may include enhanced functional capacity, improved quality of life, increased abdominal endurance, hamstring flexibility, and upper-body muscular endurance.
- **Practice and Patience:** Remember, Wall Pilates is an enjoyable and inclusive full-body workout suitable for everyone. Be patient and compassionate with yourself throughout your journey. With dedication, time, and guidance from a skilled instructor or studio, you'll master Wall Pilates, opening doors to endless opportunities for progress and advanced exercises. Additionally, practicing Wall Pilates has been linked to improved overall well-being, including increased happiness.

Embarking on a fitness journey is an exciting endeavor, but it's crucial to approach it with a well-thought-out plan. Setting realistic goals is the first step on this path. Break down your ultimate fitness objectives into smaller, achievable milestones. By doing so, you not only create a clear roadmap but also maintain a high level of motivation as you celebrate each accomplishment along the way. Remember, Rome wasn't built in a day, and neither are strong, healthy bodies.

Consistency is the linchpin of progress in your fitness routine. Regular, dedicated effort yields results over time. It's essential to establish a workout routine that you can stick to without frequent stops and starts. The journey to fitness is more of a marathon than a sprint. Avoid the temptation to increase the intensity or duration of your exercises too rapidly; a gradual, steady approach is often more effective and less prone to injury. Aim to incrementally increase your workload by no more than 10% each week.

It's perfectly normal to experience feelings of discomfort when you first start exercising. Shortness of breath, sweating, and muscle soreness are all part of the process as your body adapts to this new challenge. Embrace these sensations as signs of progress, and don't let them discourage you. Also, working out with a friend can be a powerful motivator. Not only will you enjoy the company during your sessions, but you'll also feel accountable to someone else, making it less likely for you to skip a planned workout. Having a workout buddy can transform exercise into a social and enjoyable experience.

Never underestimate the importance of warming up before your workout. Failing to do so can increase the risk of injury and reduce the effectiveness of your session. So, consider your body's natural rhythms and this sits true even when scheduling your workouts. Some people thrive on early morning sessions, while others find their energy peaks later in the day. Choose a time that aligns with your natural inclinations, as it will make it easier to stick to your routine.

Remember, throughout your fitness journey, you may encounter setbacks or moments when your motivation wanes. These are entirely normal experiences that every beginner faces. Instead of letting them discourage you, view setbacks as opportunities for growth and renewed motivation. Willpower is your greatest ally; with determination and persistence, you can overcome any challenge that comes your way on the path to a healthier, fitter you.

To conclude, Wall Pilates is more than just a fitness regimen; it's a holistic approach to health and wellness that empowers women to connect with their bodies, build strength, and enhance their quality of life. As you continue your Wall Pilates journey, remember these principles and insights to make the most of this transformative practice. If you like this book and have benefited from it, it would mean the world if you could leave us a review. Work hard, work smart, and get the results you've dreamed of, get the results you deserve.

Printed in Great Britain
by Amazon

53052126R00055